P9-DFG-897

"Whether ministering to moms who are easily triggered with their kids, or encouraging husbands and wives who are triggered in their marriages, Amber Lia faithfully has reminded us that TRIGGERS = OPPORTUNITIES! And now (cue the confetti) Amber challenges us to consider our food triggers, because triggers = opportunities here too. Each time we are tempted to turn to food as our comfort or reward is an opportunity to remember Jesus' invitation: 'Come to me, all you who are weary and burdened, and I will give you rest.' What if your hunger pangs aren't about physical hunger at all but an invitation to develop a spiritual appetite for God? If food is your trigger, this is your opportunity!"

Wendy Speake, author of *The 40-Day Sugar Fast* and coauthor of *Triggers: Exchanging Parents' Angry Reactions for Gentle Biblical Responses*

"Rather than a quick fix or trendy fad, *Food Triggers* goes deeper, all the way down to our *why*. Are you looking for real change? This book will help you start on a lasting journey toward health, inside and out."

Kirsten Oliphant, author and writing coach

"At my most desperate moment, Amber was there to gently guide me into a life-changing journey to better health. Having her as my health coach has truly been a gift."

Melissa M., client

"Amber Lia is the real deal, period. This book will free up a lot of people—believers and nonbelievers. Millions of us are battling with the same thing: our health! Amber gives us all the tools, yes, but the most powerful thing she gives is hope."

Jamil Frazier, keynote speaker, transformational coach, and bestselling author

"*Food Triggers* is a must read for anyone who is looking to uncover why they struggle with weight loss and food issues. This book is encouraging, motivating, and will help you discover ways to have a healthier relationship with food so you can live longer, have more energy, and look better."

Dr. Magdalena Battles, Doctor of Psychology

"Amber's guidance and spiritual support has allowed me to get my life back!"

Janie C., client

"*Food Triggers* covers many of the mindset and spiritual struggles that Kiersten and I battled when we both had over a hundred pounds to lose. If there's one thing we know, the truth, the practical help, and the spiritual encouragement in these pages is going to help set people free!"

Nick and Kiersten Lavallee, certified health coaches

"Amber is the friend and guide you want as you journey into a healthier life. And this is the book you want on your shelf—within reach when the celebrations, failures, and stresses of life tempt us to turn toward food. There is a better way, and Amber gently leads us to it."

Rebecca Smith, author of *A Better Life*
and founder of Better Life Bags

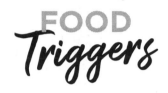

FOOD
Triggers

FOOD
Triggers

Exchanging Unhealthy Patterns for God-Honoring Habits

AMBER LIA

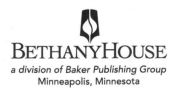

BETHANYHOUSE

a division of Baker Publishing Group
Minneapolis, Minnesota

© 2022 by Amber Lia

Published by Bethany House Publishers
11400 Hampshire Avenue South
Minneapolis, Minnesota 55438
www.bethanyhouse.com

Bethany House Publishers is a division of
Baker Publishing Group, Grand Rapids, Michigan

Printed in the United States of America

All rights reserved. No part of this publication may be reproduced, stored in a retrieval system, or transmitted in any form or by any means—for example, electronic, photocopy, recording—without the prior written permission of the publisher. The only exception is brief quotations in printed reviews.

Library of Congress Cataloging-in-Publication Data
Names: Lia, Amber, author.
Title: Food triggers : exchanging unhealthy patterns for God-honoring habits / Amber Lia.
Description: Minneapolis, Minnesota : Bethany House, a division of Baker Publishing Group, [2022]
Identifiers: LCCN 2021036349 | ISBN 9780764240591 (casebound) | ISBN 9780764238888 (trade paper)
   | ISBN 9781493435746 (ebook)
Subjects: LCSH: Dinners and dining—Religious aspects—Christianity. | Food habits. | Habit breaking—
   Religious aspects—Christianity. | Food—Religious aspects—Christianity.
Classification: LCC BR115.N87 L53 2022 | DDC 241/.68—dc23
LC record available at https://lccn.loc.gov/2021036349

Unless otherwise noted, Scripture quotations are from the Holy Bible, New International Version®. NIV®. Copyright © 1973, 1978, 1984, 2011 by Biblica, Inc.™ Used by permission of Zondervan. All rights reserved worldwide. www.zondervan.com

Scripture quotations marked DARBY are from the Darby Translation of the Bible.

Scripture quotations marked ERV are from the HOLY BIBLE: EASY-TO-READ VERSION © 2014 by Bible League International. Used by permission.

Scripture quotations marked ESV are from The Holy Bible, English Standard Version® (ESV®), copyright © 2001 by Crossway, a publishing ministry of Good News Publishers. Used by permission. All rights reserved. ESV Text Edition: 2011

Scripture quotations marked GWT are from GOD'S WORD, a copyrighted work of God's Word to the Nations. Quotations are used by permission. Copyright © 1995 by God's Word to the Nations. All rights reserved.

Scripture quotations marked THE MESSAGE are from THE MESSAGE, copyright © 1993, 2002, 2018 by Eugene H. Peterson. Used by permission of NavPress. All rights reserved. Represented by Tyndale House Publishers, Inc.

Scripture quotations marked NASB are from the New American Standard Bible® (NASB), copyright © 1960, 1962, 1963, 1968, 1971, 1972, 1973, 1975, 1977, 1995 by The Lockman Foundation. Used by permission. www.Lockman.org

Scripture quotations marked NKJV are from the New King James Version®. Copyright © 1982 by Thomas Nelson. Used by permission. All rights reserved.

Scripture quotations marked NLT are from the Holy Bible, New Living Translation, copyright © 1996, 2004, 2015 by Tyndale House Foundation. Used by permission of Tyndale House Publishers, Inc., Carol Stream, Illinois 60188. All rights reserved.

Some names and details have been changed to protect the privacy of the individuals involved.

This publication is intended to provide helpful and informative material on the subjects addressed. Readers should consult their personal health professionals before adopting any of the suggestions in this book or drawing inferences from it. The author and publisher expressly disclaim responsibility for any adverse effects arising from the use or application of the information contained in this book.

Cover design by Dan Pitts

Published in association with Books & Such Literary Management, www.booksandsuch.com.

Baker Publishing Group publications use paper produced from sustainable forestry practices and post-consumer waste whenever possible.

22 23 24 25 26 27 28   7 6 5 4 3 2 1

To my amazing clients
who are on this journey with me toward optimal health,
and for everyone who longs to believe they
can change their habits once and for all.
Let's live life to the full, together!

Contents

Your Turning Point Starts Here

When wealth is lost, nothing is lost; when health is lost, something is lost; when character is lost, all is lost.

Billy Graham

On my personal health journey over the years, a big part of my angst as a Christ-follower was the thought that if I was godly enough, I wouldn't be struggling so much with my food triggers. I felt that along with my lost health, my character must be lost too. For too long, I allowed the enemy to confuse me.

I remember how it felt to be the heaviest I had ever been. I was unhealthy and I knew it. Even though I loved Jesus and was involved in lots of ministry, I felt a deep conviction that I was out of control with my mindless eating and unhealthy pattern of craving ice cream and desserts every night. I was miserable. The quick sugar fix or carb binge left a lasting and obvious impact on my life—and one look in the mirror told the truth.

Here's what I want you to know, right at the start of *Food Triggers*: **It's possible to be in a good place spirturaly, but to not be perfect.** The enemy was trying to whisper that I was a fraud because I had no self-control regarding food and sugar. He toyed with my mind that I could do okay for a while, but that I would go right back to my old ways again. It took several starts and stops for me to finally learn how to respond correctly to my food triggers. God understands this. He knows we are not perfect. Only Jesus is perfect!

My weakness did not mean I was worthless.

It did not mean I was a fraud.

It did not mean I would never change.

It just meant I was on a spiritual journey with ups and downs. It meant I was human and still sinned, even though God had done a lot of transforming work in my life already. It meant that my weakness gave all the more glory to God because I couldn't do it on my own. This is just as true for you as it is for me.

So I didn't give in to the feelings of hopelessness when I hit rock bottom. I didn't believe I could never get a handle on my spiritual weakness and tendency to run to food. I didn't listen when Satan whispered that my food triggers were more powerful than my God.

> It's possible to be in a good place spiritually, but to not be *perfect.*

Instead, I found a medically designed plan and began eating healthy foods to help me get back on track again—and that was the practical piece I had to invest in with my time, money, and commitment. I adopted new, healthy habits *for life.* But it was mostly a spiritual transformation for me. The physical weight came off—sixty pounds—but the spiritual weight of my gluttonous tendency has been the most freeing! Facing my food triggers, one by one, was the jump-start I needed to set the stage for a lifetime of healthy habits.

Whatever plan you use to get healthy, the biggest factor for all of us is to exchange unhealthy patterns for God-honoring habits. It's foundational to remember that our weaknesses are not a reason to feel shame. They are a reason to place our hope in something bigger and better than ourselves—our faith in God.

For you, dear friend, let this book and this time of self-care be a time when lies about who you are and what you are capable of—even lies about God—fade away. Let this be a season when you learn to awaken hope that God is who He says He is. That He can and will help you in all your weaknesses. That every one of us can change when we pray expectantly and invite the Holy Spirit to transform us. That even though it may take time, nothing is impossible with God!

I am living proof of this holy exchange:

> But he said to me, "My grace is sufficient for you, for my power is made perfect in weakness." Therefore I will boast all the more gladly about my weaknesses, so that Christ's power may rest on me.
>
> 2 Corinthians 12:9

I'm betting that since you picked up this book, you have had enough of the ups and downs of getting healthy and staying healthy. I imagine that even if you have figured out a lot of your food and health issues, there is still that one thing that keeps gnawing at you. It may be that thinking about food and dealing with your health problems is exhausting you. It's taking up way too much space in your brain and messing with your emotions! No matter what plan you have used, the same old triggers trip you up. You are not alone.

Years of research and hundreds of conversations with men and women all over the country have formed the foundation for this book. The thirty-one common food triggers that we're going to talk about aren't just triggers; they manifest as shackles. It's become clear that our enemy, the devil, has thousands, if not millions, of us trapped in the bondage of unhealthy thinking and eating. I understand. My own journey from obesity to optimal health has been one that I wanted to experience in private. But God had other plans. When you find freedom and you live among captives, you can't help but want freedom for them too. *For you!*

It's possible that some of you holding this book are ready to throw off those unhealthy patterns. You are full of excitement, and the thrill of hope is coursing through your body as you prepare to dive in over the next thirty-one days. The daily discipline of reading one chapter a day over the next month will solidify your commitment to improving your health—mind, body, and soul. This is your moment!

For others, we know we need a change, but we still feel timid about proceeding. We wonder, *Is this one more thing I will fail at?* I understand your wariness.

I have had a number of life moments that are personal measures of achievement for me. At ten years old, I stepped onto the first-place block after a gymnastics meet. As an adult, it's been an immense honor to write several bestselling books. Being a mom counts as one of the best parts of my life! But perhaps one of my greatest blessings has been my journey away from unhealthy patterns and toward God-honoring habits—and helping others do the same. Now we get to take this journey *together*.

For all my little victories, my life has been peppered with far more failures. Far more "nos" than "yeses." Far more valleys than mountaintops. I don't believe I'm unique in this. My hunch is that you have had your own set of highs and lows in life. For many of us, the highs and lows affect our health—mentally, emotionally, physically, and spiritually.

Whether I was achieving my life goals or facing disappointments from one letdown or another over the years, my food triggers were the one constant. I knew the right things to do, but I often felt powerless to do them.

The apostle Paul describes the battle within us this way:

> But I need something *more*! For if I know the law but still can't keep it, and if the power of sin within me keeps sabotaging my best intentions, I obviously need help! I realize that I don't have what it takes. I can will it, but I can't *do* it. I decide to do good,

14

but I don't *really* do it; I decide not to do bad, but then I do it anyway. My decisions, such as they are, don't result in actions. Something has gone wrong deep within me and gets the better of me every time.

It happens so regularly that it's predictable. The moment I decide to do good, sin is there to trip me up. I truly delight in God's commands, but it's pretty obvious that not all of me joins in that delight. Parts of me covertly rebel, and just when I least expect it, they take charge.

Romans 7:17–23 THE MESSAGE

Have you felt any of this? As a certified health coach, I have heard this struggle verbalized from men and women of every age and stage of life, all over the world. I've come to realize that our circumstances or our food triggers don't get the final say in our personal growth. I've seen the sheer joy and relief of clients who have finally traded in their old ways and are living life to the full as God intended. Their health struggles were the portal through which they learned to succeed in areas of their lives beyond their health journeys.

When I began to apply biblical principles to each food trigger in my own life, everything changed. You see, no matter what is happening in our lives, our physical and spiritual health need not fluctuate with the ebb and flow of life's circumstances. **The spiritual tug-of-war to exchange unhealthy patterns with God-honoring habits is the ultimate food fight.** But I'm in your corner. More important, almighty God can help you achieve a new, healthier way to live.

You will hear more about my health journey throughout this book, but I want you to know, here in the beginning, that every food trigger we face has spiritual implications. Yes, when we exchange unhealthy patterns for God-honoring habits, we detox from sugar and processed foods. Yes, we lose weight and get off medications. But we also go through a spiritual transformation.

My recommendation is that you read one chapter a day for thirty-one days. Once you have completed the book, every chapter can stand alone—a sort of resource guide for revisiting specific food triggers as needed for future readings and encouragement. We will cover external food triggers—issues like traveling, holidays, our culture's obsession with large portions, and those who try to sabotage our efforts to get healthy. We will also expose internal food triggers—factors like stress, emotional eating, and loneliness or boredom. Each chapter ends with a heartfelt prayer based on Scripture, to help us connect more deeply with God.

These damaging old patterns don't have to weigh us down—or show up when we weigh in on the scale. The key to any temptation—any trigger—is to resist and then turn toward a new, healthier way of thinking and behaving. Together, we will break free from the cycle of frustration and pain that has trapped us for too long.

It's been years now since I came to the end of my rope, obese, tired, and frustrated. I faced a turning point. Slowly but surely I confronted my many food triggers, armed with the truth of God's Word and full of hope that I was at a final crossroads when it came to my health. I have never looked back.

Today can be your turning point. Through the pages of this book, I'll be with you on this journey, but take a moment right now to invite the Holy Spirit to join you too. Ask God to open your heart, unlock your understanding, and empower you with self-control, patience, strength, and hope. He will answer. With each trigger, we will expose an old pattern we need to exchange for a God-honoring habit. In so doing, we won't just get healthy bodies, we will receive spiritual health for our souls!

External Triggers

The triggers we discuss in this first section are some of the most common ways that outside obstacles hinder us from getting healthy. We will cover triggers such as traveling, holidays, our culture's obsession with large portions, and how to handle the people in our lives who should support us but don't. These external triggers don't have to steer us off track if we are aware of them—and if we apply practical biblical thinking and approaches to overcoming them.

one

When Your *Why* Is Front and Center

I couldn't remember the last time my husband, Guy, and I had celebrated Valentine's Day. In recent years, we have made date nights a priority and enjoy dining out together once a month or so, but on February 14, we typically skip the hoopla. This particular year, we decided to mark the occasion with lunch at one of our favorite steak houses. All was well until we were seated in a cozy little nook near the back of the restaurant. As I slid into the booth, my stomach grazed the table. My cheeks flushed with embarrassment. How did I get to the point that I couldn't easily slide into a booth or sit comfortably at a restaurant? How did my body become so thick that there was virtually no space between me and the table? Why had I allowed myself to get to this point?

I was on the cross-country team in college. I was even named Intramural Athlete of the Year my senior year. But even then, despite my athleticism, I carried excess pounds—mostly because I ate whatever I wanted. I might have looked somewhat fit, but I certainly wasn't healthy. After graduation, I finally took my food issues seriously. By the time I met my husband, I had been a focused recreational bodybuilder for years. It was my daily habit to run three miles in the hills around my home. I knew all the things about good nutrition and exercise. I took my health seriously and I felt great! On a spiritual level, I felt relief that I was stewarding my body and not giving in to gluttony or excess as I had been prone to do during my teen and college years. Those days were a journey toward wellness that I accomplished over the course of time. As I considered how I had gone from fit to flabby, I realized that it, too, was a journey. Thinking back, I tried to remember when I last felt in control of my health.

In 2007, I married Guy, and during the next ten years I had five pregnancies. Early on, the baby weight came off fairly quickly, but with each new child, plus a miscarriage, the struggle to lose weight increased. It felt like my metabolism was stuck and the methods I used to get back in shape when I was younger were not as effective as they once were. But I wasn't the only one feeling unhealthy. My husband packed on sympathy pounds right along with me over the course of my pregnancies. **Becoming unhealthy didn't happen overnight. I knew that getting healthy again wouldn't either.**

That evening, after our special Valentine's lunch, I felt disgusted with myself. I had to admit that I was feeling sluggish and tired most days. Keeping up with my four active sons was a challenge. I didn't just feel discouraged over the reflection in the mirror; the discouragement was multilayered as feelings of failure swept over me. I pictured each of my kids, and my heart dropped. I was not being a good example to them. The punishing sentiments continued through my mind. *What kind of Christian am I when everyone can see that I don't have self-control? How can I be so casual about the sin of overeating in my life? Why is no one calling me on it?*

I knew I needed a change. I could not keep doing the same old things and expect a better result. I had to do something different! Romans 12:2 puts it this way:

Do not conform to the pattern of this world, but be transformed by the renewing of your mind. Then you will be able to test and approve what God's will is—his good, pleasing and perfect will.

I needed to begin my health transformation by the renewing of my mind. I'm betting you do too. The pattern of the world around me was to mindlessly indulge in food. Overindulging in food and drink wasn't a topic I heard being addressed very often, even though recent estimates indicate that 42 percent of Americans are obese.[1] That's 137.4 million U.S. adults! God calls us to listen to something much more significant than our bellies. **We need not allow the growl of our stomachs to drown out the whisper of the Holy Spirit, calling us to freedom from the bondage of food.** He asks us to listen to—and live out—His will for our lives. Anything that is sinful in our lives is outside of God's will. Spiritually speaking, I believe that my issues with my health and my lack of self-control were also preventing me from living life to the full! My low energy, bulging waistline, and achy joints were simply symptoms of being outside of God's plan for my life. I knew that practically speaking, I could put down the fried chicken, but I needed the Holy Spirit to change me from the inside out.

> We need not allow the growl of our stomachs to drown out the whisper of the Holy Spirit.

I began to pray, asking God for the next steps He wanted me to take. I was sick of being a statistic. That's when I remembered my friend Tammie.

Tammie and I met more than ten years ago at a parenting class at our church. Similar in age and lifestyle, she had also gained a lot of weight over the years. Thanks to social media, we stayed in touch when we both moved to different cities, busy living our lives. Except I had been watching Tammie over the last year as she lost eighty pounds. Desperate, I reached out to her.

When we first talked, she asked me *why* I wanted to lose weight. My answers were familiar. They were some of the same reasons she chose to get healthy too. I laid out my *why* for her:

I wanted to feel pretty and enjoy shopping for clothes again.

I longed to feel energetic and free from brain fog.

I wanted to be healthy for my kids so I wouldn't cut my life short, robbing them of their mother as they grew up.

And most important, I felt convicted to break the spiritual chains from the food triggers in my life so that I could honor God with my body, which the Bible describes as the Holy Spirit's temple.

This last *why* is one I believe many Christ-followers feel immense guilt over. First Corinthians 3:16–17 says, "Do you not know that you are God's temple and that God's Spirit dwells in you? If anyone destroys God's temple, God will destroy him. For God's temple is holy, and you are that temple" (ESV). We know that being overweight is one way that we can harm our bodies. Our health matters to God. Because our bodies are a temple where God dwells, we show Him honor by treating our physical bodies well and with respect and reverence.

In my first book, *Triggers: Exchanging Parents' Angry Reactions with Gentle Biblical Responses*, coauthored with Wendy Speake, I address the guilt we sometimes feel when we fall short of God's standards for godly living:

> There is a big difference between guilt and conviction. One is meant to condemn you, the other to free you. How do you know if you are feeling an unhealthy guilt versus a righteous conviction? Guilt defeats. Conviction catapults—towards spiritual growth and freedom! God always convicts us with a loving reproach that causes us to want to keep going in His strength and not in our own flesh. It moves us forward toward growth in our spiritual lives, instead of backwards or inwards towards discouragement.[2]

Right now, some of my own personal struggles may resonate with you. You may feel frustrated with yourself. Ashamed. Stuck. But what good does it do to beat ourselves up? That's what Satan wants. He is not our friend. He is our enemy, seeking "to steal and kill and destroy" our lives (John 10:10). Instead, we get to acknowledge our areas of sin and weakness to a loving Father who is for us! God promises to cleanse us from all unrighteousness when we confess our sin to Him:

> If we confess our sins, he is faithful and just to forgive us our sins and to cleanse us from all unrighteousness.
>
> 1 John 1:9 ESV

At any time, in any place, we can tell God that we have sinned over the issues of food and our health. He will forgive us! He does not condemn us or treat us as our sins deserve. For that reason alone, my desire to honor Him with my body became a foundational *why* that has helped me to make better choices, one food trigger at a time.

Each of my *why*s was a springboard for change. And now, as an independent certified health coach myself, I know that our *why* is foundational to our long-term success.

Within weeks, Guy and I joined Tammie on a nutrition plan that fit our busy lifestyle. Early on, I knew it was an answer to prayer for us. Within just a few short weeks, our metabolisms were running as they were designed to run, our bodies finally detoxed from sugar and processed foods. Within the first few weeks, the brain fog lifted, we slept better, and the pounds were releasing from our bodies. We didn't lose them—we never wanted to find them again! We faced food trigger after food trigger head-on—the unhealthy patterns that sabotaged our health—and exchanged them for God-honoring healthy habits. As you work through your own food triggers with me in the pages of this book, you will be able to do the same, finding hope and victory no matter your age or stage in life.

Here in this first chapter, it's important for each of us to reflect on our own personal *why*. The *why* behind your decision to face and overcome your food triggers is deeply personal. Every action you take has a motive. When it comes to weight loss and getting healthy, some of us want to look better in family portraits or fit back into the clothes we wore two years ago. Maybe we want to stop snoring, have higher energy, or get off diabetes medications. Perhaps we want to achieve a bucket-list item such as completing a charity marathon or going on a vacation that requires a level of fitness we don't currently enjoy. Some of us are simply tired of quick fixes and want to commit to long-term health. Getting healthy is also a spiritual issue for many of us— just as it is for me. Knowing our *why* and keeping it front and center both clarifies and motivates us to stay on track when the going gets tough.

Picture yourself achieving your *why* for a moment. How does it make you feel? What kinds of activities are you doing? What are you wearing? Who is with you?

Keeping that visual in mind will go a long way to helping you achieve your health goals, because the food triggers will come. They are constantly all around us, often confronting us when we are at our most vulnerable. Whether you are addicted to sugar, or you simply come last on the list of priorities after taking care of your family, or you eat to comfort yourself from the discouragements you face in life—whatever the food triggers are for you—you no longer have to give in to them! We are not powerless, destined for tomorrow to look just like today! Take Philippians 4:13 (NKJV) to heart:

I can do all things through Christ who strengthens me.

Do you believe that? I do. Guy and I are living proof. God would not call us to a healthy lifestyle if it weren't possible. We can learn to exchange patterns we have allowed to rob us of feeling our best for healthier habits. We can go through a drive-through and order a salad or a lettuce-wrapped chicken burger. We can politely turn down dessert at our mother-in-law's house and we can stop grazing mindlessly from our children's dinner plates. We can commit to walking our dog in the early morning hours and we can put ourselves to bed at a decent hour. We can begin to see our *why* fulfilled!

What is *your* why? Keep it in your mind's eye as you read each of the next thirty chapters. Give your *why* to God and invite Him to face your food triggers with you. Every time I felt weak as I was pursuing my own health journey, the first new habit I established was to pause and remember my *why*. Visualizing myself playing soccer with my boys or wearing a little black dress on the next Valentine's Day as I slid into a booth with room to spare was a strong motivator. Picturing my life free from the constant struggle of overeating and laying down my sin of harmful indulgence at the feet of Jesus, leaving it there with Him so I could walk away free from that bondage, made things like drinking more water and learning healthier recipes a much easier choice for me to make.

Your *why* will motivate you.

Your *why* will inspire you.

Your *why* will stabilize your emotions.

Your *why* will focus you.

Your *why* will enable you to make good choices when temptations come.

Food triggers no longer control us when we think about our *why*. Take your health back, friends. Each meal is an opportunity for victory! Whether your *why* is a simple desire to lose a few pounds, or a longing to feel relief from the constant thoughts about food that flood your mind, you are on the right track this very moment. Your *why* will make the difference between falling back into unhealthy patterns, or finally, once and for all, embracing God-honoring habits *for life*.

Let's Pray

Lord, You are my ultimate why. I want to honor You with my body. You have given me the privilege of being Your temple, so please help me to be honorable with my eating habits. God, I need Your help. I confess that I have not been doing what is right, and I ask for Your forgiveness. Thank You for being faithful to forgive me and for helping me on this health journey. I come to You now with happy expectation for the good work You will do in me. In Jesus' name, amen!

two

When You Feel Defeated Before You Start

Wait. What?" Justin balked. "I need to drink eight 8-ounce glasses of water a day?" I assured him that was, indeed, the goal.

I could hear the wind deplete from his sails. Justin wasn't getting anywhere close to that amount of hydration, and the idea of drinking that much alarmed him. He wasn't at all sure he could do it. I could sense his mind teeter-tottering on the other end of the phone line. He imagined his failure before he had even begun—ready to hit the ground with a thud of defeat on day one of his health journey.

"I have forty pounds to lose; I'm sure I can get there by my fortieth birthday in May!" Jenna assured me. It was already the end of March.

She would need to lose almost six pounds a week to reach her goal. The odds were not in her favor if she wanted to do it safely and with the long-range goal of keeping the weight off for good.

Unlike Justin, she imagined victory before she had even begun—ready to soar toward her goals.

So, which is better? To be a Justin? Or a Jenna?

Perhaps that is the wrong question. Harvard research documents that 83 percent of the population of the United States do not have goals, and yet goal-setting typically yields a success rate of 90 percent.[1] The right question, then, becomes, *Have I set a goal for myself in the first place?* The first step toward success is not necessarily to make a reasonable goal, but to be a person who makes a plan to begin with. Justin and Jenna were *both* ahead of the game because they were willing to set goals. If you are reading this book (and you are, of course), then you are already on the upswing of success because you most likely have a goal—or at least an initial desire—to get healthy in a way that will encourage you spiritually.

We know that goal-setting is valuable, but the hard part is deciding on what goals each of us can actually achieve. Studies show that the most effective goals are ones that are outlined mindfully, are measurable, and are attached to a specific time frame.

In Justin's case, the known daily recommendation is sixty-four ounces of hydration a day, so the goal we set for him is a solid one. Drinking those eight glasses a day is not only measurable, but it's also possible to accomplish over the course of twenty-four hours. In his mind, it wasn't necessarily easy, but that part we can take in stride, as long as it's a healthy goal that has the potential for success. One day at a time, Justin can make progress, even achieving six daily glasses until his body begins to adjust. This quick, measurable progress will also motivate him to keep going toward his ultimate goal of eight 8-ounce glasses. By making a series of smaller, attainable goals along the way, we won't bite off more than we can chew.

In Jenna's case, her goal of losing more than six pounds a week for seven straight weeks doesn't fall under the recommended guidelines of a healthy weight-loss rate for most individuals. The Centers for Disease Control and Prevention (CDC) recommends losing one to two pounds a week as a healthy target.[2] What do you imagine will happen to Jenna's motivation if she is aiming for six pounds a week, only to lose three or even the recommended two pounds? She may fall into the erroneous trap of believing that it's not worth it to keep trying since she couldn't possibly reach her goal in time for her birthday bash. She may very well feel defeated by the end of week two and quit altogether, resigned to returning that little black dress she bought in the hopes of fitting into it for her party. Now she's sabotaged a worthy goal of getting healthy for life, not just for a onetime event.

As believers, we don't want to be characterized by all talk and no action. Getting healthy is a perfect opportunity to live this out. There are two practical things you can do to help you achieve your health goals:

1) Write them down.

I encourage my clients to write down their goals, and I'll encourage you to do the same. Take a moment to think about what you want for yourself. After carefully considering these goals, write them down and post them in your office, on your bathroom mirror, or in a screensaver on your phone. This way, your goals don't fade into the background of your memory or get lost among all the other things you have on your mind. They are front and center, taking priority!

2) Share them with others.

Be brave and share your goals publicly. Doing so increases your chances of success. When we put it out there, we feel a healthy pressure to follow through on our goals. That healthy pressure motivates us to stay on track. Does that make you squirm a little? Don't worry what others may think. What other people think of you is none of your business! Our friends and family will come alongside us and support us toward our goals, and those who

don't—well, that's not really our problem, but theirs. And
if we worry that we are setting ourselves up for criticism
if we don't progress, just consider this an opportunity for
personal growth. Your healthy mindset has no room for
doubts. Shove them aside and think positively!

Some of the goals we focus on within our healthy community
are getting at least seven hours of sleep every night, drinking sixty-
four ounces of liquid every day, and limiting caffeine to the morning hours. We promote engaging in regular intervals of healthy
motion several times a week and eating smaller meals every two to
three hours. We also advocate community, making a point to talk
with or interact with others who are like-minded in their desires
to achieve a healthy lifestyle. Personally, I set a goal to listen to
at least two podcasts a week that promote wellness and personal
development skills. I even set a new goal recently to take off my
makeup before bedtime. I know it's good for my skin, but I was
being lazy about it. I took the time to write the goal down and set
out my skincare products so they would be visible at night before
bedtime as a cue to put this habit in place.

In my sophomore year at college, I joined the cross-country team
on a whim. Living in the dorms and adjusting to cafeteria food took
me from a pudgy high-schooler to an even pudgier undergrad, and
I thought the forced exercise at practice might help me keep the
pounds at bay.

Our team was not exactly competitive, so I easily secured a
spot, despite my lack of ability.

Even now, I can feel the nerves and nausea that overpowered me
when I think back on that first cross-country race. The gun fired,
and we were off! I knew I wouldn't be first to finish the course,
but I wasn't prepared for the blow that came when I crossed the
chalk line. I came in last place. *Dead last!* I vowed I would never
be last again . . . and I wasn't. Every subsequent race, I bettered
my time by a minute here and a minute there. My mindset was

no longer to place but to simply be faster than the girl behind me until I completed the last ragged, wobbly, exhausted stride over the finish line.

Though I never became competitive—or svelte—I finished the season and managed to stave off the dreaded weight gain I feared, even though I wasn't being mindful of proper nutrition. The most valuable lesson of running cross-country, however, was the concept of endurance that burned deeply, with every gasping breath, into my mind. I learned what it meant to persevere when your legs feel like they cannot possibly take another step, much less propel your body forward. I managed to face the hills that loomed before me when everything in my mind told me to stop. I learned how to track the next curve in the path with my eyes laser-focused on going just a little bit farther, a little bit faster.

I have to admit that one of the main reasons I didn't quit was because I had an audience. My teammates, friends, and even perfect strangers were witnesses. I wasn't about to stop running with all those people watching! When we live out loud, showing others that we are in the race to better our health, a little bit of healthy peer pressure can be good for us! We don't want to be crippled by what others think of us, but I believe there is a balance we can achieve when we invite others into our process. Another added benefit is that it allows us to inspire those who are still on the sidelines. If we can do it, maybe they can too!

My experience as a runner made Philippians 3:13–14 a favorite passage that has encouraged me through various seasons of life:

> Brothers and sisters, I do not consider myself yet to have taken hold of it. But one thing I do: Forgetting what is behind and straining toward what is ahead, I press on toward the goal to win the prize for which God has called me heavenward in Christ Jesus.

We have already established that God wants us to steward our bodies well and to be healthy in mind and body. Taking care of our health is one way we obey God, one way we live life to the full, one way we receive His blessings. For me, having a healthy body means I get to stay in the race! It's my way of saying, *"Lord, I'll do my part to do all I can to serve You for as long as I can."* We may not be able to mitigate all of life's challenges, but we can certainly do what is within our power to improve our health. Goal-setting is a simple and practical step toward the prize of good health and the even more valuable eternal prize of honoring God in all that we do.

Some of us are hesitant to set goals now because we have failed to meet them in the past. Persevering in good works will require us to forget "what is behind" as we look to the future. F. Scott Fitzgerald reminds us, "You mustn't confuse a single failure with a final defeat."[3] The former can become a stepping-stone, the latter a gravestone over our hopes and dreams for a better life. The past does not define the future. It sets us up for the future that our good God has prepared for us, if we embrace it! **Failure is a wonderful teacher. We learn how to do things differently next time—and that's a good thing!**

After that first cross-country race, I learned the art of pacing myself with another runner. I set a meeting with my coach to talk about how to manage the cramping I experienced during that grueling first race. I took that initial failure and learned from it. The next race was only a little bit better, but each time I improved, because my goal mattered to me. I did not anticipate a first-place medal, but my goals were attainable, and each next mini victory encouraged me toward the next one.

> **Failure is a wonderful teacher. We learn how to do things differently next time—and that's a good thing!**

When I look back at that season of my life, I am prouder that I did not allow a last-place standing to stop me from carrying on, than if I had been a star runner. I don't think I'd feel the same satisfaction if I had actually won a first-place medal! The value of persevering has stayed with me over the years, while a ribbon around my neck would certainly fade over time. Maya Angelou writes, "You may encounter many defeats, but you must not be defeated. In fact, it may be necessary to encounter the defeats, so you can know who you are, what you can rise from, how you can still come out of it."[4]

In chapter 1, we talked about your *why*. Hopefully you still have it front and center in your mind. Your *why* serves several purposes on your health journey. Not only is it foundational for beginning, but it also propels you through obstacles you face along the way. I like to think of our *why* as an acronym:

When

Hindrances

Yield

When challenges come, remembering your *why* forces hindrances (the things that might trip you up or trigger you) to yield, opening up a pathway to success. The desire to eat emotionally becomes less desirable as you ponder your strong need to reduce your dependency on medications. The impulse to flop on the couch after work becomes less magnetic when you visualize keeping up with your buddies on the basketball court. *Your hindrances yield to your why!*

My friend and client Marley is a professional baker. And I mean, a real pro. She bakes magnificent artful concoctions day in and day out. Her social media feeds are filled with cakes that look like unicorns, dinosaurs, motorcycles, and succulent gardens. Her world, day in and day out, is an edible art studio. The health of this busy mom and wife took a backseat for a lot of years. She was doing well on a plan, losing weight and feeling great. But then it got hard. She started straying from eating the things that were helping her and not being as mindful. The scale stopped moving in the right direction. With more than one hundred pounds to lose, she still had quite a journey ahead of her. I called her up via video chat and listened as she shared her current reality. Marley felt a little deflated and unmotivated to keep up with her new lifestyle, though she desperately wanted to lose the weight and get her life back.

"Marley, do you know what to do to get healthy, and can you do it?" I asked.

"Yes, absolutely," she quickly replied.

"Okay. So, you can get healthy. That's one option. What is the other option? What would happen if you don't get healthy and lose this weight?" I questioned.

Looking straight at me, she paused for only a moment through the computer screen. "I'll die," she said.

Both of us let those heavy words have their moment. I felt the goose bumps rise on my skin, and my heart dropped. She was right. Marley decided right then and there to get back on track and continue to get healthy. She knew that she was in a life-or-death situation. The magnitude of what was at stake became a *why* that allowed the hindrances and triggers she was facing—baking, busy schedules, lethargy—to yield to her desire to **live**. Each of her kids is her *why*. Wearing more comfortable shoes is her *why*. Being able to go on vacation and wear a regular seat belt on the plane is her *why*. Prolonging her life and sustaining longevity is her *why*. Living is her *why*! Are her confections impressive? Yes. But her willingness to overcome obstacles and create her best life is sweeter than anything she creates in her kitchen.

Sometimes, as powerful as our *why* is, we can ignore it. This is why we write it down and keep it visible, along with our goals. Fight for your *why*. Protect it. Nurture it.

Now it's your turn. You have your *why* defined and visible. Here at the start of this book, set two or three mindful, measurable, and attainable goals that are motivated by your *why*. Write them down. Share them with others. Consider that you may very well need to persevere, recalibrate, or refocus as you journey, but stay in the race. Remember that this process is about personal growth, learning from what is working and what is not, and being willing to keep taking the next step toward success. Because really, just as Marley considered, what is the alternative? I don't believe for one minute that you picked this book up because you want to stay stuck. That you want to let your food triggers have the last say. Those days are behind you. Defeat is an option, but not for you. Your *why* is strong, your goals are worthy, and your God is present and able to help you in your time of need. This is where your hindrances yield. This is where you finish the race. This is where you prize your health, and your health becomes the prize.

Let's Pray

Lord, help me to do the next right thing. Help me to achieve reasonable goals, day by day, so that I don't give in to defeat. Help me to remember that the past is the past. This is a new day with new opportunities to run the race You have set before me. Thank You, Lord, for running alongside me and never giving up on me. I see my hindrances yield to Your good plans for my life. Keep me focused, one victory at a time. In Jesus' name, amen!

three

When You Are Bored

I had never felt more bored in my life. Or more guilty. All I wanted to do when I grew up was what my mother had done: get married, have kids, become a homemaker. I waited much longer than I thought I would for those dreams to come to fruition, but now that they were reality, I felt like a caged animal, trapped in my little house in the small beach town on the central coast of California that Guy moved us to with our two young sons. I loved my children enough to die for them, but the day-in, day-out tedium of wash, rinse, repeat as I cooked and cleaned over and over again felt uninspired and heavy. I loved being a mom, but I did not love my life—or the feelings of guilt for not being complete and content with where God had me.

After several months of feeling stuck in this woebegone mood, I determined to pull myself up by my bootstraps and get on with life. Make it what I wanted it to be. Take charge! Instead, my efforts were squashed. I took the boys on long walks to parks and attempted to set up playdates with other moms I met in town or at church. Most of the time, people had other things to do. I felt like my brain cells were dying for lack of adult conversation. I wasn't just feeling a bit bummed. Discouragement settled into my bones. I had no idea I could be so delighted with my children as they discovered the world around them, and yet so totally bored with the regularity of my own life at the same time. Sadly, that frustration led to feeling triggered in my parenting, and those triggers led to anger. The boredom mixed with anger led to eating. Since there wasn't a lot to do in my small town, I tried my hand at gourmet cooking and some baking. Well, somebody had to eat the baked goods, and not too many people were knocking on my door, so I "volunteered." But I still felt unfulfilled—and a lot puffier.

More than a year went by, and one day, when I sent Guy off to work, I had a moment of clarity as I closed the heavy coffin of a door behind him. I sensed the Holy Spirit whispering to my heart. I felt courage well up in place of my feelings of boredom and frustration. God was going to help me so that I did not give in to my flesh any longer. I sensed a new path of purpose opening up before me.

Every day when my kids took a nap, I committed to short periods of reflection and prayer. I opened my Bible and began to dig in to verses about anger, frustration, hope, and purpose. I remembered a favorite book, *The Purpose Driven Life*, and the words that first struck me many years ago as Rick Warren boldly drew the bottom line with the first pages of his book:

> It's not about you. The purpose of your life is far greater than your own personal fulfillment, your peace of mind, or even your happiness. It's far greater than your family, your career, or even your wildest dreams and ambitions. If you want to know why you were placed on this planet, you must begin with God. You were born *by* his purpose and *for* his purpose.[1]

Life wasn't about me. I forgot this in the midst of my routine as a stay-at-home mom. I forgot that everything I do, whether I eat or drink, can be to the glory of God (1 Corinthians 10:31). My life was turning inward upon itself, and because we are made in the supernatural image of God, we can never be satisfied by mere flesh (or food). It wasn't that my life wasn't interesting enough, it's that I didn't value the meaningfulness of that which I had deemed meaningless. Furthermore, because my eyes were turned inward toward my internal problems, I couldn't see the potential for new things God was orchestrating in my life—like laying the foundation for transformation toward gentle parenting (which would become the subject of my first book in a line of many).

I suspect that you, like me, may eat because you are bored. You are bored by your job. You are bored by your office space, your neighborhood, your commute, your friends, your hairdo, your daily needs. Your current routine feels too . . . *routine*. Those things that once excited you have become as tarnished as a worn penny. The luster, lacking. And I suspect that like me, you are bored because you forgot your purpose. Or your *potential*.

There in that quaint little house just down the dusty street from town, the Lord looked me square in the eye through His Word, day by day, and lovingly convicted me that I was wasting the good life He had blessed me with. I was harming my body with overeating as a way to scratch an incessant itch that could never be satisfied with blueberry muffins or a leek gratin. **The instinctive desire we all feel to live life to the full cannot lie dormant. It will always find a manner in which to present itself.** It will either present as a healthy, vibrant mindset and the fulfillment of a God-centered calling, or it will attempt to manifest in other more temporary and often harmful outlets—like addiction to food, shopping, or alcohol. **Pick your poison. Or find your purpose.**

The overhaul I needed didn't occur on day one. At first, God worked on my parenting. Then He worked on my marriage. Then He worked on my diet. I'm not going to tell you it was always easy. In *East of Eden*, John Steinbeck wrote, "It is a hard thing to leave any deeply routined life, even if you hate it."[2] Routines have power. The thing about habits is that when they are healthy ones, we become forces for good in our own lives and in the lives of others. But when they are unhealthy habits, the routine can ruin us.

How, then, do we determine our ultimate purpose? Foundationally, it's in our relationship with Jesus. Second, it's by understanding that we don't always need to figure out every detail of our lives *today*. Instead, we can begin by knowing that God has it all planned out for us:

> It's in Christ that we find out who we are and what we are living for. Long before we first heard of Christ and got our hopes up, he had his eye on us, had designs on us for glorious living, part of the overall purpose he is working out in everything and everyone.
>
> Ephesians 1:11–12 THE MESSAGE

Glorious living. That's how we should describe our lives! Each of us plays a part in the grand design of God's plan for humanity. You are an important part of a grandiose whole. Please don't think I'm suggesting that every moment of our lives is one big ball of kinetic excitement and awe-inspiring interactions, one after another. That's not real life. But when we find ourselves in the center of God's will, doing the next right thing, even something as simple as eating and drinking, or cleaning and scrubbing, becomes meaningful. **Mundane routines that enable supernatural callings are as meaningful as the grandest accomplishment.** Writing this book is a perfect example. The fulfillment of finishing the last page and hearing from readers who are encouraged and impacted by my books is delightful. Editing and crafting endnotes or citations, waking in the darkness to write when I might prefer to slumber on, not so much. Still, the nitty gritty does not dismay, because it's a part of something bigger than me—a calling to help others. To love my brothers and sisters by spurring them on toward love and good deeds, page by page.

God didn't place us here for us to take up residence, eating and drinking and sleeping, and then repeat. He created us for good works—and as Christ-followers, our lives should be lived on the edge of the supernatural. How could we think that settling for boredom—and boredom eating—could possibly be a suitable choice for the princes and princesses of the kingdom? We were made for so much more than that! There is a pattern we can outline when we think about boredom eating:

Life feels dissatisfying. Dissatisfaction leads to a *desire*.

Option 1: The desire is healthy and leads to stepping into more of what God planned for your life.

Option 2: The desire is unhealthy and leads to something temporal and ultimately feeds the dissatisfaction even more.

When we hunger for a thing that never satisfies, it takes on the form of a drug—or an idol in our lives. God has strong words for such a state as option two. For those of us who love God, we are considered His friends. And yet Paul describes enemies of Christ as those whose lives are spent on their "appetites":

Their end is destruction, their god is their belly, and they glory in their shame, with minds set on earthly things.

Philippians 3:19 esv

It's a rather sobering thought that I, someone who loved the Lord, was behaving like someone who exhibited the same behaviors as His enemies. My god was my belly. And it didn't look, or feel, good. As I leaned in to my quiet times during those early days of struggle as a young mom, the truth of God's Word took on renewed meaning in my life. I began to see homemaking as a gift.

We started hosting dinners for families from church and looking for ways to serve others. My husband began to hint that I should start a blog, and I did. That blog led to books. I wish I could say that I immediately got a handle on my boredom eating, but that, too, took time. Slowly but surely I began to exercise and eat right. Eventually, with several more pregnancies, my weight would rise and fall, but the trap of eating from boredom did not plague me as it once did.

Only after I took the time to acknowledge that I was not living life to the full, appreciating the blessings of my life, just as it was, did possibilities open up to me.

I'd like to ask you, Why do you eat *what* you eat? Why do you eat *when* you eat? What in your life is not working for you? Is food serving you or suffocating your emotions? Food is fuel. If we use it for anything else, and we are overweight or obese, then we need to examine whether we are using food as a drug or using food as a dietary benefit as it was intended. There is a big difference.

Here are some telltale signs you might be using food as a drug to satisfy that which cannot be satisfied by food:

You think about food often throughout the day. (**Here's a thought: Do you think about the pleasures of food more than the pleasures of being a Christ-follower?**)

You hide food or hide when you are eating food.

You look forward to holiday foods more than what the holidays signify.

You make excuses for your obesity.

You feel momentary delight when you are eating, but afterward, you feel sick and discouraged.

You buy mostly processed foods and food that is high in sugar. You justify this by saying it's less expensive.

You have full pantries but little fresh foods in the refrigerator or vegetable bin.

For me, coming to this realization about myself was not easy. But it did feel strangely empowering. I don't want you to feel shame. Shame is not from God. I want you to feel hopeful. When we can pinpoint one of our food triggers, like boredom eating, we have a starting point that can lead us to positive change!

Let's put in place a few healthy habits that will help us shift from boredom eating to eating and living with purpose:

1. Clean out your pantry. If an item on your shelf has more than four grams of sugar in the ingredients list, toss it in the trash. (Yes, I do advocate "wasting" food that is unhealthy. Don't pass it on to others. If it's not good for us, it's not good for our neighbors either. Junk food is not nutrition!)

2. Stock your fridge with healthy snacks. Some of our favorites: dill pickle spears, baby carrots, sugar-free Jell-O, celery sticks, mini peppers, whole-grain bread, low-fat Greek yogurt, berries, and low-fat cheese.

3. Fill up on spiritual bread and milk before physical food. Take the time to have your quiet times with God every day. Listen to how His Word guides your steps. Ask Him to reveal to you your purpose.

4. Identify your talents and pinpoint your interests. What are some things you have always wanted to do? (There are lots of helpful books on determining your gifts.)

5. Examine the times of day when you turn to boredom eating the most. Now replace that activity with something healthier. If you normally snack after the kids are in bed while you watch TV, go brush your teeth and put a "Closed" sign on the kitchen cabinet or refrigerator to remind you that you don't need to keep eating.

Let's begin to consider what better use we can make of our time to combat boredom eating. Our church has been seeking partners to help in the Spanish-speaking ministry. I'm betting your church has a time slot you can fill to help fold programs or pray over prayer request cards. Just the other day, I realized I had a stack of gently used clothing I could take pictures of and post in an online group for moms who might benefit from having them. Call a friend in need instead of calling for takeout. If boredom eating signals a lack of purpose, then it's time to green-light ways we can be a blessing to others. Turning a temptation into a testimony of God's work in our lives is one way to ensure victory in this battle of the bulge.

Not every season of life is filled with excitement. And yet it's easy to get into a routine that drains our enthusiasm for life and the world around us. When we feel unfulfilled, we turn to food to fill the gap and placate our boredom. What can we do to fill our days with meaningful work and relationships? How do we break the habit of being triggered by boredom? I'm convinced the answer is living a more vibrant life, just as God desires for each of us. There's nothing boring about committing, here and now, to making the most of our lives. What aids us in that goal is not found at the bottom of the ice cream carton. It's found in the wake of a heart on fire, fueled by purpose and ignited by hope.

Let's Pray

Dear God, thank You for creating me for purpose. I know that life has its moments when I need to persevere, but help me to turn my boredom into bondage-breaking moments of victory. Help me to replace the unhealthy pattern of boredom eating with the God-honoring habit of spiritual growth. I don't want to waste my life. Thank You for giving me purpose, even in the routine moments of my day. In Jesus' name, amen!

four

When Your Clothes Don't Fit and You Can't Hide It

As soon as Sean sat down, he tugged on his shirt and crossed his arms. Every. Time. Even when his arms went numb, he sat stiffly, attempting to hide the bulge around his middle.

The few pictures Melanie allowed to be taken of herself were group pictures—with her face peering over the shoulders of others while she stood concealed in the back.

Carolina had the habit of crossing her ankles, attempting to give the illusion that her thighs were not as big as she perceived them to be.

Everyone thought Neil was just a hipster with his long hair hanging over the sides of his face, but for him, his hairstyle gave him a place to hide. Yes, there is power in the words we say, but many of us communicate far more by our body language.

I can see myself in Sean. I vividly remember my mother asking me, as a pudgy preteen, why I always had my arms folded across my middle. I wasn't brave enough to put to words what was in my heart. I was keenly aware of the little roll that appeared when I sat down—and I did my best to conceal it. My twelve-year-old arms, dotted with freckles, became a straitjacket. The problem was that instead of communicating my insecurity, my mom interpreted my body language as sullenness. I wasn't just struggling with the extra weight I carried, but the weight of being misunderstood bore heavily on my heart as well. **My body language communicated a message I was not intending to send.**

As a young mother, I turned into Melanie. You won't find me in front of my family photos from 2015 to 2018. I'll never get those years back—or the opportunity to show what was true and honest about me. I hid my exuberant, joyful personality by standing in the background. How about you? Are you a Carolina? Or a Neil? Is your body language communicating inadvertently to others that you are shy or sullen? Do you realize that when you're so ashamed of how you look, you become the warden of a prison of your own design? But as all prison guards do, *you* hold the keys to freedom.

When I think about the people I love most, I think about the freedom I want them to feel in every area of their lives. It's one of the things I love about taking my kids to a park or a playground. They run off ahead of me, gleefully flinging arms wide open, unconscious of how they look, ready to experience all the opportunities for fun and frivolity before them. Their eyes light up in anticipation of making new acquaintances. They swing their legs up and over the monkey bars, hair standing on end, feet dangling. They don't dwell on how their clothing feels or if they are shouting too loudly. They are free! Immersed in wild abandon and unchained from inhibitions. What is it about adulthood that causes us to care more about what others think of us than the pleasures of embracing who we are? I recognize that maturity brings with it a new sense of decorum, but listening to our insecurities and then acting on them moves us from decorum to hesitancy, embarrassment—and reluctance. None of these states of being is reminiscent of living life to the full, the ideal that is laid out for us in Scripture.

Freedom is a core need within the human DNA, designed by God. In John 8:36, we find these beautiful words: "So if the Son sets you free, you will be free indeed." The ultimate freedom is found in relationship with Jesus Christ, who came to free us from the chains of sin and death. At its core, this truth sets us up to experience the ripple effect of God's grace in our everyday lives. Our eternal destiny secure, our everyday lives are now ripe with the promise of freedom in every aspect. Free to trust that others will accept us just as we are. (And if they don't, well, at least we know the truth about them—and it's always best to know the truth.) Free to accept ourselves—strengths *and* flaws. Free to believe that God loves us overweight, underweight, or somewhere in between. Free to acknowledge that perhaps we have unhealthy habits, but we have a desire to change.

One of the greatest writers of all time is Danish storyteller Hans Christian Andersen. In reviewing *Hans Christian Andersen: A New Life* by biographer Jens Andersen, British journalist Anne Chisholm writes, "Andersen himself was a tall, ugly boy with a big nose and big feet, and when he grew up with a beautiful singing voice and a passion for the theater he was cruelly teased and mocked by other children."[1] His famous tale *The Ugly Duckling*, published in 1843, has been a favorite children's story for generations and is steeped in popular culture.

The story goes that a swan's egg rolled into the nest of some ducklings. Upon hatching, the wobbly gray swan is rejected by his nestmates—lovely-looking ducklings who mock him and cruelly mistreat him. They repeatedly tell him he is ugly, and soon he believes them. Cartoons of this cherished story show the duckling, head down, wings slumped, with a tear-streaked face, wandering from lake to lake, never fitting in with those around him. He notices a herd of beautiful swans, but it's not until a year has passed and he sees his own reflection in the lake—with snow-white feathers and his elegant neck—that he realizes he is the object of beauty he admired in others. Joining a herd of wild swans, he spreads his wings and embraces his identity with joy.

46

Andersen speculated that he might have been the illegitimate child of the prince of Denmark, who one day became king. It seems that *The Ugly Duckling* is a metaphor for his experiences growing up.

Sadly, not much has changed in humanity in the nearly two hundred years since Andersen's tale was written. **We still put a high mark on appearances. We judge books by the cover instead of by the Good Book.** The Bible cautions us against putting too much emphasis on how we or others look. In the book of 1 Samuel, God is appointing the next king of Israel, the lowly David. Samuel mistakenly believes that God will choose Eliab, who is tall and pleasing to the eye. But God warns Samuel,

> "Do not look at his appearance or at his physical stature, because I have refused him. For the LORD does not see as man sees; for man looks at the outward appearance, but the LORD looks at the heart."
>
> 1 Samuel 16:7 NKJV

I confess, I still instinctively cross my arms when I sit down. Some habits die hard. It's comforting for us to know that our appearance does not dictate our purpose or our value in the eyes of God. If our jeans are too snug or our boots won't zip over our calves, it may mean we have some work to do in the area of healthy eating, but it's not an opportunity to beat ourselves up. I wonder how many of us have the words of our "nestmates" still reverberating in our ears. The pattern of listening to criticism, remembering the unkind words of those who called us "ugly ducklings" firmly entrenched in our subconscious. Or even the seemingly harmless scrutiny of others. I can still picture myself standing before my mother, unnerved and embarrassed.

The freedom from such damaging scripts lies in replacing them with truth.

When we have a biblical view of our appearance, our body language shifts. Our message shifts. The warden's keys rattle in the lock, and freedom looms in front of us. Has our unhealthy pattern been to feel ashamed of our bodies? To listen to the voices of others—or our own—that tell us we are not pretty enough? Handsome enough? Accepted? Do we cross our arms and curse our appearance? Biblical habits are healthy habits. God tells us not to look at appearance or physical stature as a means of worth or suitability. We must examine our hearts—and invite God to do the same:

> Search me, God, and know my heart;
>   test me and know my anxious thoughts.
> See if there is any offensive way in me,
>   and lead me in the way everlasting.
>   Psalm 139:23–24

Our self-consciousness is the snuffer that Satan uses to dim the light God asks us to shine. Satan wants us to feel miserable and look it. Who in the world would be drawn to that? And that is his underworldly aim. Recognizing these body language behaviors is the first step toward allowing God to work in our hearts so that we can become comfortable in our own skin and make the most of the kingdom work God has for us to do. Pray this prayer along with the psalmist. Ask God to help you let go of your insecurities and give you the courage to believe your value and worth are equal whether the scale is high or low, your thighs thick or thin, your ankles swollen or slim.

Interestingly, swans typically know their limits when it comes to eating, and do not overeat.[2] We have a lot to learn from our feathered friends, and we will address practical ways to avoid overeating in future chapters. I believe God wants our bodies healthy, but we must begin with a healthy mindset. A godly mindset. You are not an ugly duckling. Genesis 1:27 says, "So God created mankind in his own image, in the image of God he created them; male and female he created them." You were created in the very image of almighty God, and everything He does is good.

If the tire around our middle reflects some measure of our sinfulness or weakness, it does not reflect our value. And yet the image staring back at us in the mirror (or on the pond's undulating surface) is also meant for freedom—freedom from sin and the shackles of valuing the wrong things, like other people's opinions or our own wrong scripts. It is said that swans are highly intelligent, remembering who has been kind to them and who has not.[3] Perhaps there have been many careless words from others that have been less than kind to us. Dwelling on those memories will not serve to help us move forward. Let's remember those who have been kind, and especially the kindness of the Lord. **Your body language is far too powerful to waste on your insecurities.** Today, stand a little taller. Step from behind the crowd in the portrait. Uncross your arms and your ankles. Cut your hair. Unfurl your body from shame, and shine as you are meant to.

Let's Pray

Dear Father, You don't want me to think less of myself, but You do want me to think of myself less often. When I feel insecure, Lord, be my security. Help me to communicate Your openness and love by the way I carry myself. I don't want to feel self-conscious any longer. Thank You for reminding me that I am made in Your image and that You accept me just as I am. In Jesus' name, amen!

five

When You Lack Portion Control

You are not to blame. Yes, I know. You are the one lifting the fork to your mouth, but right from the start, I want you to understand that in the food war, we have been unequally armed. We have slowly, one meal at a time, become overweight, fighting our food triggers with an inadequate armory. We come to the table hungry, and therefore, vulnerable. We also come unaware that the battlegrounds have been staged without our knowledge. We thought we were just on a dinner date with friends. Our vulnerability and our ignorance have worked against us for a long time. We scoot our chairs up to the table and politely place our linen napkin on our laps. And then the assault—the onslaught—begins.

We didn't really even see it coming. It was disguised in alluring aromas, plated with confident hands by a woman or man wearing an authoritative white chef's hat. We assumed that what we got is what we *should* get. Little did we know that nine in ten U.S. restaurants are serving meals that exceed the recommended calorie limit for a single meal, sometimes more than *twice* the 570 calories some experts recommend an average adult woman consumes at lunch or dinner. (And for men who regularly dine out, the recommended daily average of 2,400 calories puts them equally at risk when regularly dining out.)[1] This alarming statistic related to restaurants describes only our entrees. It doesn't include alcohol, beverages, appetizers, bread baskets, or dessert.[2] Can you imagine the calorie count of a meal with all those typical components?

Proverbs 23:2 says, "Put a knife to your throat if you are given to gluttony." Yikes. Those are some strong words. *The Message* paraphrase of this verse warns not to "gobble your food, don't talk with your mouth full. And don't stuff yourself; bridle your appetite." I often felt conviction about my weight because I valued my identity as someone who is organized and disciplined in most areas. My bedroom is tidy. Financially, I am not an overindulgent spender. When it comes to juggling work and home life, I have been able to find a rhythm—a workable balance. But take one look at my eating habits, and I was out of control. I gave little thought to the aftermath of my unhealthy pattern of consuming larger-than-recommended portions of food.

It's been said that when we know better, we do better. The conflict we face when we battle our cultural norms is more easily won when we awaken to reality. All of us can assuage this food trigger by getting practical. Checking the menu for the restaurant before we arrive and deciding what we will order in advance is how we fortify our resolve to get healthy and stay healthy. When the server offers us bread, we smile and say, "No, thank you." When they ask if we would like a soda, we ask for seltzer water with a splash of lemon—in a fun martini glass. *Thank you very much*. We choose an entree of lean protein, prepared with minimal cooking oils or butters, with a side of steamed or roasted vegetables. We order salad dressing on the side. If our lettuce-wrapped burger is bigger than our fist, we cut it in half and take the rest home—or send it happily on its way with our dining partner. **We remind ourselves that** we have had cheesecake before. **We know what it tastes like. We can skip it this time. And next time too.** Instead of dwelling on what we are not having, we enjoy all the things we *are* having—fuel for our body, a serene dining experience in a pleasing environment, and the blessing of fellowship with others. Yes, when we know better, we do better. Think better. Choose better. Eat better. Live better!

Not long ago, I found some old pictures of when I was at my unhealthiest. At five feet five inches, I weighed 215 pounds. My obesity made me groggy and fatigued. I told myself I was just working too hard, but that wasn't the reason I felt like I was walking through sludge every day. One glimpse at my neck, bulging and swollen with excess fat, and I cringed. It wasn't out of pure vanity. I cringed at the thought that I had been kidding myself into ignoring what large portions of food and binge eating had done to my body. It's been said that gluttony is not a secret vice. I might have been lying to myself, but the pictures told the truth.

In many ways, our culture has brainwashed us with massive portions and helpings that are, well, NOT helping. Gluttony has become acceptable. One meal at a time, we have allowed bigger to be better. When I began measuring the recommended serving sizes on packages of my favorite snacks, the reality of how mindless I had been with my helpings hit hard. I wondered why I had simply been opening a bag and reaching inside all these years. If I'm honest, I think I didn't really want to know. I wasn't in the habit of checking those portion sizes, and it took some health scares and the need to buy a bigger jeans size to wake me up. If you feel frustrated by this battle for portion control, I understand. I have been there.

In 2020, the world came to a standstill as it had not done in a hundred years. COVID-19 spread like wildfire across the globe and turned our lives upside down. I remember a feeling of panic at the onset of the pandemic. Like many, I stockpiled as many canned goods and toilet paper rolls as I could. Whenever I went to the store or tried to place an online order, I ordered more than I needed for that week. After doing so over the course of several months, I noticed that I had begun to live with a scarcity mindset. A need to hoard that didn't break easily. It unsettled me. As a mother, I wanted to make sure my family had what we needed. An internal, nurturing "mama bear" prowled the aisles, hunting and gathering. Even when things returned to normal at the grocery store, the pattern was hard to break. My mindset had been conditioned for overkill.

This uncontrollable pull to gather more than we need is not new. In Exodus 16, the Israelite nation was miraculously led out of Egypt by Moses, passing through the Red Sea on dry ground and following a pillar of fire by night and a cloud by day, leading them to the eventual Promised Land. Not long into the journey, a mere two months, and they began to grumble against Moses and his brother, Aaron:

> The Israelites said to them, "If only we had died by the LORD's hand in Egypt! There we sat around pots of meat and ate all the food we wanted, but you have brought us out into this desert to starve this entire assembly to death."
>
> Exodus 16:3

Of course, we know that God had no intention of leading them into a desert to starve—they were His chosen people destined for a chosen and decadent land flowing with milk and honey. In their petulance, God provided. He told them that at twilight, they would eat meat, and quail filled the land for them to gather. And in the morning, a cracker-like sustenance called manna was scattered on the ground. God used Moses to instruct them concerning this provision. The Israelites were to gather only a portion—an omer—for each person in their tent. No more, no less. But just like me at a Trader Joe's during a pandemic, some of them did not trust the Supplier:

> However, some of them paid no attention to Moses; they kept part of it until morning, but it was full of maggots and began to smell.
>
> Exodus 16:20

Wouldn't it be nice to have automatic portion control as the Israelites had? Perhaps not. Wandering for forty years in the desert because of their sin was no small discipline. Still, the life we live when we are overweight can feel just as stagnant and dreary as forty years in a wasteland. The price we pay today takes us on a different sort of journey, one that leads to diabetes. Heart disease. Cancer. High blood pressure. The United States Department of Agriculture is tasked with helping us understand the price we are paying for our own unwillingness to listen. According to the USDA's latest dietary guidelines, "It has become increasingly clear that diet-related chronic diseases, such as cardiovascular disease, type 2 diabetes, obesity, liver disease, some types of cancer, and dental caries, pose a major public health problem for Americans. Today, 60 percent of adults have one or more diet-related chronic diseases."[3] Each year, obesity-related medical costs total hundreds of billions of dollars.

Sadly, this pattern has been ongoing for the last twenty-five years, as more than half the adult population is overweight or obese. We are well on our way to a forty-year stretch of turmoil in our own land. The enormous financial and personal price we are paying is something that I personally am no longer willing to contribute to. Portion control is a key element in healthy eating, but so many of us have been unwitting consumers.

Early on in my quest for less, I began to study portion recommendations on the back of packages of foods we brought home from the store. We did simple things to combat overeating, like leaving measuring spoons and cups out on the countertop and teaching our kids to measure a single serving of their snacks into a bowl, instead of eating from a bag by the handful. We bought smaller plates for dinnertime so we did not overdo helpings. We don't squirt condiments from a container—they go from bottle to measuring spoon to burger. We began sharing entrees when we ate out and leaving leftovers behind. Imagine if we became mindful and intentional in this way and then taught the next generation to do the same!

I said it before, and I'll say it again. We were not to blame for our ignorance. But now we know. Now we are empowered and able to turn the tide, one serving size at a time. The generous portions we have been eating have stolen our health. In giving us temporary pleasure, they have robbed us of long-term satisfaction. The war for the health of our country and our world is magnificent in size, but it is not insurmountable. Our willingness to make small changes can make a big impact. Let's fight the good fight as we arm ourselves with the knowledge that bigger is not better. **Each time we measure our meals, we do immeasurable good for our health.**

Let's Pray

Lord, I know—I know I'm eating portions that are not healthy. The culture's influence is strong, but it is not stronger than my desire to get healthy. Father, thank You for opening my eyes to how often I overeat. Help me to adjust spiritually as I adjust physically so that I do not hunger or thirst for anything but You. In Jesus' name, amen!

six

When Your Doctor Tells You to Lose Weight Before It's Too Late

Your doctor just prescribed yet another medication to get your cholesterol under control, or maybe she has warned you that if you don't lose weight, you are at risk for diabetes. I get it. We aren't always ready to take the plunge and change our eating habits, even though intellectually we know we should. While it's true that no one can do the work of getting healthy for you, others can act as a trigger to spur you toward being a good steward of your health. That shove in the right direction can come in the form of a health coach or personal trainer, but many times, it's by health scares. Nonetheless, that shove may be just the ignitor you need to get healthy for good.

"Too late." Those are words tinted with regret, aren't they? It's one thing to be too late for a train or a bus—we can always catch the next one. But what if we get to a point in our health where it truly is too late? For most of us, that would mean our lives are about to be cut short. But if your doctor has told you that you need to lose weight, it's not too late to make changes. Let's not gloss over that statement. One of my greatest sorrows as a health coach is hearing of the loss of life from someone who decided to wait to get healthy, only to succumb to their preventable disease. For some it was too late, but for you, it is not.

In the months leading up to 2020 and before COVID-19 became a reality, 83 percent of men and 72 percent of women were projected to be overweight or obese by the start of the new year.[1] Let that sink in for a minute. That means our society has both conditioned and *condoned* our food triggers instead of exchanging them for God-honoring habits. If you and I decide to go against the flow, we will be a rarity!

My husband fit into that statistic for many years. At forty-eight years old, Guy was more than sixty pounds overweight and taking cholesterol medication. I was worried about him. One fine fall day, he came home from his annual health checkup with a prescription for blood pressure medications in hand. My heart was gripped in fear at the news. Guy's dad passed away from a sudden heart attack when Guy was right out of college. He spent his adult life without his father to commiserate with and mentor him. I never got to meet my father-in-law. Pulmonary issues ran in his family history. I knew that if Guy didn't get his weight under control, our sons could have the same sorrowful experience of growing up without a father figure in their lives, and I might miss the chance to grow old with my best friend.

I also knew that I could not get healthy *for* Guy. He had to do it *for himself*. Thankfully, he recognized that things were not going to get better or easier if he didn't make some changes. We both realized that the health issues he was facing were preventable if he shed the extra pounds. In a matter of six months, Guy lost the weight, and he has kept it off ever since. His daily dose of medicating is now a thing of the past.

If you have ever left the doctor's office with your own diagnosis, you understand that feeling of fear. Guy and I were both statistics before we started facing our food triggers, and maybe you are too.

According to studies from 2009 to 2012, every third child in the U.S. from age two to nineteen was overweight or obese. Cardiovascular disease (CVD) affected about 84 million men and women twenty years and older.[2] That's 35 percent of the population—and that rate has steadily risen year by year!

I'm not a numbers girl, but these next statistics took my breath away. In 2020, the CDC revealed that 34.2 million people had type 2 diabetes. An astonishing 7.3 million people who met the laboratory criteria for having diabetes were not aware they had it. An even scarier revelation is that 88 million people eighteen years or older have prediabetes.[3] That's 34.5 percent of the adult U.S. population. The CDC also states that those who are obese are also at risk for mental illnesses such as clinical depression, anxiety, and other mental disorders.[4]

When I look at these overwhelming numbers, it feels hopeless. I long to see a change in our world for better health, but how can you or I possibly make a dent in the lives of millions of people? The food and pharmaceutical industries are powerful, and we are just little fish swimming in a big stream. Then I remembered something I once heard a pastor say: "Do for one what you wish you could do for many." Do you know who that "one" is? It's me. It's you. As I researched diabetes, the CDC made one prominent admission: The alarming rate of diabetes and obesity in our children is related to patterns they see in their families. When I decided to get control of my health, this realization was a central push for me in the right direction. I knew I did not want my four precious boys following my poor example. I did not want them to struggle in their health the way I was struggling. The way Guy was struggling. Impacting my own family's health was something I could control. Influencing the legacy of the Lia family was within my grasp if I could release us from the deadly grip of our obesogenic world.

Diabetes isn't the only concern. The CDC also reports that almost 23 percent of overweight and 31 percent of obese Americans have doctor-diagnosed arthritis. According to arthritis.org, a key study published found that overweight and obese adults with knee osteoarthritis (OA) found that losing one pound of weight resulted in four pounds of pressure being removed.[5] In other words, losing just ten pounds from your body would relieve forty pounds of pressure from your knees. You may not aspire to become an Irish step dancer, but what might that relief mean to you in everyday moments like climbing the stairs or going on a walk with your friends, children, or grandchildren?

Sure, being overweight means you are part of the crowd, but it also probably makes you feel like you are missing out. Have you ever longed for something more in your life? An internal urge to do something that makes a difference? As long as I felt the dread of how I looked and felt when I was unhealthy, it made the idea of doing something more with my life seem out of reach. The fear of missing out (FOMO) was something I lived with daily. One of my favorite Bible verses is one that many claim as their favorite:

> "For I know the plans I have for you," declares the LORD, "plans to prosper you and not to harm you, plans to give you hope and a future."
>
> Jeremiah 29:11

When Guy and I considered what we were doing to our bodies by overeating, I had to compare my actions with God's desires. God desired to prosper me and give me hope. I'll never forget the feelings of disappointment and hopelessness I felt when I would open my closet door and rifle through all the dresses and pants and shirts that did not fit, or the hopelessness of battling embarrassing and painful psoriasis for years before I detoxed my body. God's plans didn't include harming me; I was harming myself with every unhealthy pattern: mindless snacking, not drinking enough water, staying up too late at night, and sitting too much during the day, to name a few. I was following a plan that would literally cut my life short if I did not exchange my unhealthy patterns for

God-honoring habits. I was absolutely missing out on God's best. That was something to be afraid of!

My favorite verse from Jeremiah was not going to come to fruition by chance. I realized that in order for God's best plans to be realized in my life, I needed to do my part. Listen, I'm not preaching a prosperity- or works-based faith here—I'm simply saying that we can do a lot to sabotage the good things God has in store for us. We can count on His faithfulness and goodness even when we are not faithful or good, but we can't lead a life of deception, or adultery, or gluttony, and expect that we won't pay the consequences. **God is a good Father, and good fathers don't let their kids run wild.** They teach and train and correct when they see problem areas with their sons and daughters. Hebrews 12:4–7 puts it this way:

> In your struggle against sin, you have not yet resisted to the point of shedding your blood. And have you completely forgotten this word of encouragement that addresses you as a father addresses his son? It says,
>
> > "My son, do not make light of the Lord's discipline,
> > and do not lose heart when he rebukes you,
> > because the Lord disciplines the one he loves,
> > and he chastens everyone he accepts as his son."
>
> Endure hardship as discipline; God is treating you as his children. For what children are not disciplined by their father?

I didn't want any more of God's discipline in my life, so I decided to discipline my body in healthy ways. **The discipline of healthy living was a far better situation than experiencing the discipline of God because of my gluttony.** It's often been said that losing weight is hard. But being overweight is also hard. Choose your hard! For me and Guy, committing to getting healthy was a hard choice, but it was one of the best choices we have ever made. In a matter of months, Guy was able to ditch the cholesterol and blood pressure medications. When I saw him making efforts to get healthy, it also awakened in me a newfound respect for my husband. That in turn made us feel more connected to one another emotionally. **Our *weight loss* resulted in a *gain* for our marriage.** I was incredibly thankful that I didn't have to worry so much about becoming a widow as a young wife and mom. Guy was doing something about his health before it was too late!

I remember a time not long ago when one of my sons had his own health scare. A mysterious and rapidly growing skin tumor appeared on his little shoulder. The doctor was concerned. We had some testing done that took several days for results to arrive. I will never forget each day we had with him during the waiting period. My heart was anxious, try though I might to leave my cares with the Lord. I didn't want to take my eyes off my boy. I worried

> The discipline of healthy living was a far better situation than experiencing the discipline of God because of my gluttony.

about whether his life was hanging in the balance, and I cherished every precious moment. We did things together that I would normally put off. I made his favorite meals. I studied the curve of his nose and drank in the sight of his floppy mop of hair. Nothing about him was taken for granted. I valued his life! I valued *him* because I loved him!

The results came back all clear, and I have never been more relieved in my life, but I have never forgotten how every moment of every day counted, when I thought we might not have had many left. It wasn't too late for us to make the most of our relationships with our boys. I've taken that to heart ever since.

Doctors and health scares can only go so far in helping us take our health seriously. We need to be willing to do the hard thing when it's an overall good thing. So let me ask, Does it matter to you? Are you a person who takes the easy path in life? Might this be an opportunity for personal growth? Spiritual growth? Now that you know better, will you do better? **Ignorance is not bliss. It's death.** Today, it's not too late. God's eyes search the whole earth, looking for those whose hearts are fully committed to Him so that He can strengthen them (2 Chronicles 16:9). Amid the billions, will He locate you? He knows your heart, and His promise is to help you on your health journey. Take Him up on the offer today so that you can experience *every tomorrow.*

Let's Pray

Dear God, You have given me life today. Do not let me take it for granted. I don't want to be a statistic, Lord. It's not too late for me. Strengthen me as You have promised, and prolong my life. Show me the patterns I need to change, and give me the courage to overcome them. I invite Your Holy Spirit to lead the way. I will follow You and not the crowd. In Jesus' name, amen!

seven

When Others Sabotage You or You Sabotage Yourself

H ey, Amber, did you know Susan is spreading a rumor that you lost weight because you probably have an eating disorder?" My head snapped around to stare at my cousin Julia. I couldn't believe what I had just heard. My friend Susan is someone I had known for a long time. She was practically family. Someone I trusted. Someone I thought cared about me. She seemed glad for me that I had lost weight. I racked my brain to understand why on earth she would make such a hurtful claim, and came up short. Instead of being happy for me, it felt like she was trying to sabotage me.

One of my clients, Faith, beamed with joy at our week-one celebration call to talk about how her first seven days on our health program had gone. She was losing weight, inflammation had receded in her hands, and her energy was high. And then she told me that her husband had been making fun of her. "Oh, here you go again, starting something you probably won't finish!" he teased.

The light behind Faith's eyes dimmed faster than the battery on an old iPhone as she shared his comments with me. My heart dropped.

Sometimes others try to trigger us into abandoning our healthy lifestyle in less obvious ways. When your mother finds out about your hard day, she runs right over with lasagna and garlic bread to comfort you. Well-meaning friends gift you with your favorite candy for your birthday. Stella was two months into her health journey and doing beautifully when she shared her success with her friend from church. Stella was excited to be making progress in an area of her life she thought would never change, and she gushed about the fact that she was finally off sugar, learning new healthy recipes, and fitting into clothes she had not worn in years. She and her friend agreed to meet up the next day to chat and visit. When Stella's friend arrived, she came bearing gifts: an iced mocha and a big slice of coffee cake. Caught off guard, Stella felt pressured to indulge in the foods she had been so successful to avoid.

In my health journey, I have surrounded myself with like-minded people. One of my mentors is Jamil Frazier. If it wasn't for him, I wouldn't have gotten healthy myself, and it's likely you would not be reading this book right now. In his book *The Twelve Shifts*, he describes a scenario where your enemy slips some strychnine (a deadly poison) into your coffee. He explains that if you didn't notice, "you would drink the coffee and die." But what if you were drinking coffee with "your mom, your best friend, your favorite cousin, and your pastor," and by accident, one of them "knocked some strychnine into your coffee, unnoticed?" The answer would be the same. "You would drink the coffee, and *you would still be just as dead.*"[1]

I hear it all the time. Clients and friends come to me bewildered by the comments and actions of those who they assumed would support them on their health journey, but they don't. Instead, they seem to be trying to sabotage them! Most likely, these friends and family members aren't fully conscious of how their words and actions are hurtful. Sometimes they bring us poison wrapped in the folds of wax paper and tied with a bow from the pastry shop.

They don't realize they just knocked strychnine into our coffee. In those cases, we do our best to educate and inform them. And possibly gain an ally. But sometimes, those close to us do not feel inspired by our success. They feel threatened by it. Instead of feeling excited for us, we are a mirror, reflecting their own insecurities and failures of the past. Caught off guard, they don't know what to do with this changed person in front of them. They feel jealous, convicted, and uncomfortable with our changes. They want things to stay the same, and the fear of how our lives are changing makes them feel like they are being left behind. They grasp for ways to keep things status quo—and in doing so, unwittingly strive to sabotage our journey and our confidence.

Justin, a new client, recently shared that he was having a hard time breaking the habit of his Sunday night football parties. His tribe of friends were drinking buddies, enjoying beer and wine as they rooted for their favorite teams. The environment was not conducive to his new lifestyle. He decided that if his old patterns—and old friends—were doing more harm than good, then at least for football season, he needed to find some new friends. He knew he needed to surround himself with buddies who were like-minded, looking to reach similar health goals. Creating an environment that would support him became one more God-honoring habit he had to put in place to reach success.

These are not easy things to talk about. None of us wants to be seen as a person who drops friends or comes across as better than others. But there comes a point when we need to communicate our needs to the people in our lives and give them the opportunity to lovingly support us or let us go. The tension of those moments is one we don't often prepare for or see coming. Your health journey will present you with hard choices, and it won't just be saying no to onion rings—but saying no to people or jobs or places that are not moving you toward God's best for you.

It's not all doom and gloom, however. Tiana knew that her family gatherings over the holidays were going to be interesting. She

65

would be spending four nights out of her safe environment, around people who were not committed to a healthy lifestyle. Already twenty pounds closer to her goal weight, she wasn't about to be swayed by her extended family. Her small crowd of aunts and uncles and cousins were big ice cream fans. Sure enough, every night after dinner, the herd headed to the kitchen counter for a nightly banana split bar. Tiana, armed with gluten-free, sugar-free brownies, quietly prepared her healthy dessert in front of them. "Mmm," she hummed as she took a small bite, savoring the simple treat as they indulged in their overflowing bowls. The next night, the pattern repeated—but with one stark difference. Only half of her relatives opted for ice cream. On night three, the dessert dash dwindled. By night four, one of her cousins asked her if she could help him get healthy too. Sharing our journey often results in a positive impact on others, so let's not let those who are skeptical or critical sabotage the good habits we have put in place. Tiana could have followed the crowd, but instead, she became an example of someone they would want to follow.

When I think about those who try to sabotage our journey or who are simply making different choices than we are, I consider Proverbs 13:20, which says, "Whoever walks with the wise becomes wise, but the companion of fools will suffer harm" (ESV). Is it foolish to binge-drink? Both science and Scripture would tell us it is. Is it foolish to keep company on a regular basis with people who tempt us to go down paths where we don't want to go? First Corinthians 15:33 has the answer: "Do not be deceived: 'Bad company ruins good morals'" (ESV).

Does that mean we instantly drop our friends and family like hot potatoes if they don't support us? Not always. When we exchange unhealthy patterns for God-honoring habits related to food, we grow in our personal development. We learn to advocate for ourselves! If you are anything like me, you don't relish confrontation or hard conversations, but being willing to communicate when friends and family are saying and doing things that hurt or hinder us is a healthy habit in and of itself. And a biblical one. Being honest and asking for what we need is always the right thing to do. Can you call your mother-in-law before your visit for Easter and share that you are eating differently in this new season of getting healthy? Would you be willing to ask if you could provide a dessert that complements your healthy lifestyle? Or bring a salad? Why not? You may gain an ally in the process. And just maybe, you will have a positive impact on them as well. They may awaken to their own unhealthy patterns and realize that you are not competition, but a companion to partner with for positive change.

The only thing worse than when someone tries to sabotage us is when we attempt to sabotage ourselves. This can take various forms: Setting foot in environments that are tempting, continuing to stock unhealthy foods in our pantry, or disregarding the help of those who seek to assist us are tools of the self-saboteur. Afraid we won't be successful, we set ourselves up for failure before we can prove ourselves right. If we have tried to lose weight in the past, only to gain it back or quit too soon, one more failure feels too scary. What will that reveal about us? That we are not good enough? Not as strong or acceptable as the next guy? But what is the alternative? We read in the previous chapter about the incredible danger that looms before us if we don't get control of our health.

There is something admirable about someone who tries, even if they fail. Setbacks are setups for comebacks. Failures are only possible for the person who didn't quit, and because failures are opportunities to learn and grow, failures serve to get us that much closer to our goals. Those who try are people who take even just a glimmer of hope and hold on to it. They are people willing to take a risk. People who don't settle for staying stuck. Those are not the qualities of failures. Those are the qualities of potential. **When you say yes to getting healthy, you say yes to becoming a person who no longer allows obstacles to overcome you. You step into your Christlike identity as an overcomer.**

In our culture, there are land mines at every turn because we live in an obesogenic world where our environment perpetuates unhealthy patterns and where poor nutrition is right around the block. Advertisements and menus beckon us to drink their poison. We unwittingly undermine ourselves when we show up at a party without healthy options for ourselves or to share with others. When most people around us are overweight or obese—as statistics show—it's easy to follow the crowd or let them pressure us to go and do likewise. But not us.

When so many things are present to work against us, allowing the people in our lives—or even ourselves—to set traps is the easy way out. God didn't design us for the easy path. John 16:33 tells us we will have trouble in this world. But Jesus encourages us to "take heart" because He has "overcome the world." Have someone's jealous words hurt your feelings? Been less than enthusiastic about your absence from the cookie party? Criticized your new look? Take heart. That kind of trouble is unfortunate, but it's far less trouble than a lifetime of obesity, disease, and discouragement from unhealthy patterns. It's not our fault when others react poorly to our transformation, but we can take responsibility for protecting our journey and measuring our success not by the comments and actions of others, but by our willingness to forge ahead, in spite of the obstacles.

Let's Pray

Father, I know that You are for me, always. Please allow my friends and family to support me, but help me to forge ahead in my health journey even if they do not. Help me to be kind and strong as I advocate for myself. It's honoring You that matters the most, and I commit to doing just that. Lord, thank You for accepting me. If I can be a positive influence on others, help me to do that too. Please ease the hurt from those who have not been supportive, and allow me to offer grace. In Jesus' name, amen!

When Community Means Food

Several years ago, Guy experienced a void in his life. As a Christian in Hollywood, feeling on the outs is a regular emotional battle. Guy had been working in film and television for many years. It's a challenging industry, and the lack of community was getting to him. He decided to do something about it, so on a fine spring evening, we worked together to spruce up our backyard in anticipation of nearly thirty men—actors, directors, producers, and entertainment lawyers—to congregate around the heat of a roaring fire overlooking the valley where we live. The idea was that I would prepare an epic homemade meal for these entertainment leaders, and they would spend time hanging out, commiserating, and praying for one another as they faced the challenges of working in an often dark and unforgiving industry. We hoped to feed their bellies and their hearts.

It was a huge success! It turns out Guy wasn't the only one in need of mentorship and encouragement. All through the evening, they stepped back and forth over the threshold from the outdoors to our dining room, hovering over our table teeming with appetizers and main courses, back and forth from table to fire pit for times of prayer and then breaks for refreshments. And thus, the "Fire Pit" was born. That evening became the first of many over the years. Those men have gone on to work together on many notable films and TV projects, seeking to honor God and entertain viewers, but the biggest blessing has been the relationships they fostered over those meals.

I admit, one of the things I loved most about meeting for Bible study or my son's preschool group at church was the wonderful homemade food that the women prepared for special events when we came together. Take a moment and think about the last team meeting you held at work or a recent after party for your child's soccer team. Was there food involved? Beverages? One of the first things I consider when having friends over is what I will feed them. Are you the same? I bet your mouth is watering even now!

All around the world, community means food. I have spent enough time living abroad to know that we are not unique. As Christians, we love to host potlucks and game nights, youth group all-nighters, and ladies' teas. God instructs us in the value of gathering and being like-minded. He designed us for community! The Bible encourages us not to neglect meeting together (Hebrews 10:25). The description of Christ-followers in the early church sounds a lot like the church in the twenty-first century:

> They broke bread in their homes and ate together with glad and sincere hearts, praising God and enjoying the favor of all the people.
>
> Acts 2:46–47

Not much has changed over the centuries when it comes to fellowship. We care and we share! We share meals, our time, and our resources from a place of love and generosity. That is a godly thing! And yet, for many of us who are only beginning to recognize that our culture has brainwashed us into believing that food's primary purpose is pleasure, not fuel, we are easily lured into decadence and overindulgence. This is especially true when our community assumes that food—often unhealthy food—is a given.

When Guy and I hosted his first Fire Pit gathering, I prepared a rich lasagna, oozing with cheese, high-fat sausage, and refined pasta. Baskets of cheesy garlic bread lined both ends of our buffet table. And I didn't stop at one dessert: I made my famous triple-layer-triple-chocolate cake and a lemon cream pie with lemons from my little backyard orchard. I was proud of my cooking! I had done it in love, but I also appreciated the compliments and wanted my husband's admiration for my hard work and skills in the kitchen. My motives weren't entirely pure. Cooking for others was in part about *me*. I wasn't concerned about my health or my husband's—though we were both obese at the time. Nor did I consider whether the meal was sustenance for the hard-working men who would eat it. I just wanted them to feel pleasure and enjoy the meal I provided.

Spiritually, this realization was an aha moment for me when I began to learn how to eat right and take care of my body. I had to acknowledge that gluttony wasn't my only area of sin that needed examination. I also had much of myself wrapped up in my motives for cooking and baking, and that had to change. Galatians 6:3 says, "If anyone thinks they are something when they are not, they deceive themselves." That was me, all right. I deceived myself into thinking I had no ulterior motives. My heart was in the right place. Sort of. But my heart can't always be trusted.

There is nothing wrong with receiving praise for a job well done, but I had made that more important than my physical well-being. I'm not willing to let any seed of pride—no matter how seemingly insignificant—reside in my heart. And so gathering in community, and the way I focused on food, involved soul searching and making room for God to search my heart.

This past year, the Fire Pit has looked much different. No longer able, in good conscience, to lay out decadent and unhealthy options for my own family, I wasn't about to serve those high carb and high calorie meals to my guests either. Nowadays, we barbecue chicken, make pots of turkey chili, and lay out a variety of vegetable trays and salads when guests come over. I have replaced the sugary pies and cakes with fruit platters and yogurt. When my in-laws came for dinner recently, after the meal we moved on to playing games. No post-meal sweets required! Of course, there are thousands of healthy recipes for desserts and other favorite meals at our fingertips online and in the many health-minded cookbooks in stores, but I tend to keep things simple. It's helped me stay humble now that I recognize the underlying pride that also presented itself when my ego was looking for affirmation. My body isn't just healthier. So is my mindset. So is my spiritual growth!

The solution to staying healthy is not to avoid community. One of my favorite verses in the Bible gives a practical picture of friendship:

> Two are better than one,
>   because they have a good return for their labor:
> If either of them falls down,
>   one can help the other up.
> But pity anyone who falls
>   and has no one to help them up.
>
> Ecclesiastes 4:9–10

Recently, a popular catchphrase has been circulating as our world navigates the aftermath of a pandemic. "We Are Better Together" is written across signage and communicated on the news, reminding us that though we are often under lockdowns, physically distanced, and asked to stay in our homes, we are still part of a community seeking to do what is best for one another. At no other time in my life have I experienced the need for gathering together more than in 2020 and 2021, when that privilege became

sidelined by COVID-19. In June of 2020, the CDC acknowledged
the toll it was taking on our community:

Overall, 40.9% of respondents reported at least one adverse mental
or behavioral health condition, including symptoms of anxiety disorder or depressive disorder (30.9%), symptoms of a trauma- and
stressor-related disorder (TSRD) related to the pandemic (26.3%).[1]

Depression and mental health issues for adults and kids sky-
rocketed during this season of isolation. We were designed by God
to be with one another and help one another. Friends are good for
our health! The Mayo Clinic highlights just some of the benefits:

Friends also play a significant role in promoting your overall health.
Adults with strong social support have a reduced risk of many significant health problems, including depression, high blood pressure
and an unhealthy body mass index (BMI). Studies have even found
that older adults with a rich social life are likely to live longer than
their peers with fewer connections.[2]

Experts tell us that loneliness can even lead to arthritis.[3] It's
clear that isolation leads to other mental health issues as well.
One study examined data from 309,000 people and found that
those "with strong relationships had half the risk of premature
death from all causes."[4] We know that being together is good
for us—as long as we don't derail those benefits by indulging in
unhealthy patterns.

Facing our food triggers is never just about food. When we strip
away the facade that food often creates, we actually make room for
the greater good. We move away from the kitchen counter and into
more meaningful conversations. Our fixation is not on whether
anyone will notice if we sneak another cookie; instead, we become
more intent on the people we are gathered with, looking for ways
to connect more authentically. **When we gather together over food,**

let the fellowship be our focus! The distraction of food no longer prevents us from awakening to the things that really matter. We remove loneliness from our lives. We feel seen and valued, and we take full advantage of the opportunity to give instead of take. This requires intentionality.

It's not just all in our heads. Studies show that when we gather in groups, we are setting ourselves up to be triggered if we are not mindful. The *Journal of Eating Disorders* explains:

> People eat more when they eat in groups. Why? It turns out that when people eat in groups, more food is available to each of them, on average. We propose that people arrange for more food to be available when they plan to eat in a group because eating in a group—at least a group of friends—makes it possible for people to eat more than they ordinarily would. Such overindulgence is one of the pleasures of group eating.[5]

If this is true, and I believe it is, how do we fight these triggers and still enjoy community? How do we navigate temptations? It's one thing to be the host and lay out platters of foods that won't sabotage our health journey, but what about when we are the guest?

Pink-sprinkled cake donuts and chocolate-glazed twists line the tables in the church lobby. Life groups meet weekly for potlucks and barbecues. Family reunions wouldn't be the same without Aunt Chika's pecan pie or Grandpa Joe's family meatballs slathered in homemade marinara. Do we spend our whole time at the party eyeballing the meatballs? Are we so distracted by the cupcakes that we miss some of the other wonderful qualities of community? I know I did. Before I broke the cycle of addiction to sugar, my body craved it. I couldn't wait for the bride and groom to cut the cake already! I didn't mind if a little spittle landed on the kids' birthday cake when they blew out the candles. I just wanted a slice!

So, let's get practical. Remember, this health journey thing can sometimes feel like a battle. Preparing for the triggers and then practicing healthy habits over time will change our lives—and our relationships—for good!

When you are planning to attend a community event, consider these practical approaches:

1. Bring your own healthy options. If you are unable to, do the best you can to eat nutritiously with what is available. **Remember that eating one meal that is not part of your plan won't erase your healthy lifestyle.**

2. Eat a meal before you arrive. This will also set you up for success if few healthy options are offered. Allowing yourself to get too hungry weakens your resolve.

3. Keep in mind you don't have to eat anything you don't want to. Peer pressure wasn't fun in middle school, so let's learn from that lesson and not succumb as adults.

4. Stand away from the food and even with your back to it. Out of sight, out of mind! Take one plate of food and then put your hands in your pockets or offer to hold cousin Rita's cute baby. When your hands are full, they are less likely to graze the food table.

5. Decide to stick with water or unsweetened tea.

6. Put a goal in place that has nothing to do with food. I like to make sure I meet at least three new people and ask them questions about their lives and interests. Instead of hanging out by the mini bar, jump in the pool with the kids or participate in the game of Frisbee golf. Try something new!

7. Attend the event with the mindset of being a blessing to others. Look for ways to serve the host or jump in to wash the dishes instead of lounging about eating a pastry or having one more scone.

8. Focus on celebrating the moment, and the people, in your community. Embrace the joy of the event itself.

9. Remember that you are an example to others. When we see friends and family making good choices for themselves, it often motivates us to do the same. **Your decision to make healthy choices impacts my decision to make healthy choices!**

10. Come away with gratitude for your ability to keep on your health journey and for the people God has placed in your circle of influence.

Learning to make healthy choices when we come together is critical in a world where community often means food. By all means, keep gathering together. Keep sharing and being generous toward one another. But let's do so without the emphasis on what we will put in our mouths, and instead on what we will give from our hearts. **Gaining community does not mean we have to gain pounds.** When we train ourselves to focus on fellowship, not the food, enjoying the experiences around us turns our community-based food triggers into opportunities for richer relationships.

Let's Pray

Dear God, I want to be in a healthy community. Change my thinking about food and help me to focus on fellowship when it's time to gather together. I hate that my thoughts are so often about food. It feels like I am missing out on more meaningful moments when I'm at a party or event. Lord, purify my motives and help me see the value in self-control. Let me be a blessing to others in moments when I feel weak so that I can overcome this food trigger and find freedom from my unhealthy patterns. In Jesus' name, amen!

nine

When Losing Weight Is Harder Than It Used to Be

A s children, we can't wait to grow up. I'll never forget my son's preschool graduation ceremony. Each child came to the microphone to share what they wanted to be when they grow up. Several sweet children talked about becoming ballerinas or firefighters. One boy impressed the audience with his desire to be a brain surgeon. My little cutie's turn was next. "I want to be a Red Robin worker!" he expressed with delight. Chuckles reverberated around the room. Of course, my son would pick his favorite restaurant as his ideal career choice—managers at Red Robin offer balloons when you finish your meal! Who wouldn't want to be the person who gets to do that all day? For my boy, it seemed like the pinnacle of pleasure.

I'm betting that, like me, when you thought about your life as an adult, you didn't consider the responsibilities and pressures of adulthood or aging. All we envisioned was the red balloons.

We didn't anticipate that our bubbles would burst. The joys of life are plenty, but along with the blessings and gifts of age come responsibilities, stress, less time to nurture ourselves, arthritis, thyroid issues, bum knees, and weight gain.

My friend Joanne and I knew each other as young girls, and now, nearly thirty years later, we compare notes on how our bodies are holding up. Committed to being healthy as we age, we can't help but recognize that it is much harder to do than when we were younger. Before we both committed to our health journeys, we compared notes on achy backs and swollen joints. We groaned over the agony of trying to lose those five extra pounds after the holidays. I noticed a significant challenge to lose stubborn pregnancy weight gain after my fourth child was born. Can you relate? Do you find that the methods you tried to lose weight ten years ago are less effective now? Are you questioning why it feels like your metabolism has slowed?

Whenever I take on a new client to coach, I do a short assessment of their eating habits and sleep patterns. Time and time again they come to me frustrated. The methods they used at one time are no longer working for them. My own health journey began that way. It seemed like increasing my exercise and watching my portions was simply not enough to have an impact as I got older. But don't be alarmed! Aging does not have to be a sentence for poor health. Not in the least.

We will cover some practical ways to rev up our metabolisms so that we can experience ultra-health and longevity, but it's comforting to note that the Bible highlights the blessings of living to a healthy old age. Moses was a man of great responsibility. God used him to lead His people, the Israelite nation, out of slavery and into the Promised Land. It was not an easy task. Over the years, he wandered in the desert, dealt with rebellious people, and was continually tasked with being God's instrument to perform miracles. Few of us will carry the responsibilities and hardships that Moses endured. And yet, his life was one of vitality right until the end:

> Moses was 120 years old when he died, yet his eyesight was clear, and he was as strong as ever.
>
> Deuteronomy 34:7 NLT

Imagine! Instead of feeling weak and feeble, there are many things we can do to combat decline. Like Moses, I pray that we will be "as strong as ever" when our last days draw near. I imagine that the impact of stress on Moses' health could have been significant, but he had a pattern of communing with God, taking his troubles to Him in prayer, and acting in faithful obedience, even when it did not make sense. The result was a man who lived life to the full, all his days.

Ultimately, God is the One who numbers our days, and we should do the same. Psalm 90:12 instructs us to number our days so that "we may gain a heart of wisdom." Imagine where you will be and how you will feel five years from now. Ten. Twenty. Fifty! Do you suddenly feel the urgency to make the most of the life you have? I do! That's wise. God gave us purpose in this life. He has plans for us to accomplish, and He longs for us to grow in relationship with Him. He has instructed us to be spiritually disciplined, developing His character in our hearts, being an example to others, and running our race in such a way that we win the prize when it is said and done. How likely are we to do all God designed for us if we are sick in bed, unable to move, or prematurely aged in such a way that we can't be as useful as we would like to be? Not very likely!

One spiritually fundamental truth of aging well is to mature well in our faith. There is a difference between just aging and aging well. We can be seventy-five years old and still be a baby spiritually. Not only do we benefit emotionally and relationally when we grow in spiritual maturity and wisdom, but God makes a direct link to our spiritual growth with physical vibrancy:

> The righteous will flourish like a palm tree,
> they will grow like a cedar of Lebanon;

planted in the house of the LORD,
they will flourish in the courts of our God.
They will still bear fruit in old age,
they will stay fresh and green.

Psalm 92:12–14

That sounds pretty good to me! Picture yourself with your grandchildren, riding bikes along the beautiful coast on a family vacation. Imagine being strong enough to carry your great-grandchild over the threshold of your door, or participating in a Thanksgiving Turkey Trot as a senior citizen. Consider how it will feel to be able to spring out of bed to make your own breakfast from the comfort of your home instead of living in an assisted living facility—and the financial peace that comes from not burdening your children with the cost of such a place. Think about the work you can do to further God's kingdom because your mind and body are sharp as you "bear fruit in old age," full of meaningful work and fulfillment in your life, instead of watching TV all day, immobile and bored.

I'll never forget Ruth, a woman in her eighties at our church. No matter which service you attended, weekly Bible study, or kids' camp, Ruth was there. Widowed for many years, she devoted her life to serving the body of Christ. Ruth could be found in the aisles as a prayer partner after services, in the kitchen filling water cups for snack time during the kids' Sunday school classes, or mentoring young moms on Friday nights. Her body kept up with her acute mind, and she wasn't the only one to benefit from her vibrant health. We all did.

If you grew up in a Christian home or attended Sunday school at church, you most likely were taught Ephesians 6:1–3: "Children, obey your parents in the Lord, for this is right. 'Honor your father and mother'—which is the first commandment with a promise—'so that it may go well with you and that you may enjoy long life on the earth.'" In our book *Parenting Scripts*,[1] my coauthor, Wendy Speake, and I highlight things moms and dads can say to kids in the heat of frustrating moments that breathe life, instead of using knee-jerk words that wound. This passage from Ephesians 6 is one of my favorite scripts to use with my children. When my son is tempted to disobey, I ask him one simple question based on this verse: "Son, what happens when you disobey?" His reply is swift because he knows things don't go well. My kids have been taught that one of the benefits of obedience in all things is that life will go well for us and we will experience a "long life on the earth." If my son disobeys me and jumps from a tall tree, he may very well be cutting his life short. At the very least, spending summer in a cast would impact the quality of his life. In the same way, all God's instructions are for our good and for our protection. When He tells us to avoid gluttony and to steward our temple well, He knows what He is talking about. **Our obedience will always give birth to blessings—and good health is just one of them!**

> Our obedience will always give birth to blessings and good health is just one of them!

Practically speaking, there are scientific reasons behind why it's more challenging to lose weight or increase our overall health as we age. Because our bodies naturally lose about 3 to 8 percent of lean muscle per decade as we age beyond thirty, if we continue on the same diet, we will gain weight. One expert explains it this way:

> Why does that loss of muscle matter? Because lean muscle uses more calories than fat. So unless you're regularly strength training with weights to maintain and build muscle, your body will need fewer calories each day. That makes weight gain likely if you continue to consume the same number of calories as you did when you were younger.[2]

Endocrinologists warn us that we must decrease our calorie intake and increase our muscle mass to maintain our health. But hormones play a role too. As women approach menopause, estrogen drops. This encourages fat to settle around the belly, and that shift in fat storage is unhealthy. We already know from previous chapters that fat storage puts us at increased risk of high blood pressure, heart disease, high cholesterol, and type 2 diabetes. Marcio Griebeler, MD, an endocrinologist at Cleveland Clinic in Ohio, notes that the decrease in estrogen also impacts our mood, making it more emotionally challenging to commit to a healthy diet and exercise. When men age, their levels of testosterone begin to drop. Because testosterone helps regulate fat distribution and muscle strength and mass, men's bodies burn fewer calories as they age as well.[3]

When I was a kid, I spent long hours practicing cartwheels outside and roller-skating in the local school parking lot. Summers were spent swimming and taking walks with my family. With adulthood comes a more sedentary lifestyle. But children today are fixated on screens while eating chips from a bag. I recently watched a TikTok video clip of one mom supporting her teenage son's gaming hobby by filling a box in his room with Swiss chocolate cake rolls, potato chips, soda, licorice, and cookies. Junk food. And yet the hundreds of comments praised her for being a supportive and fun mom. Childhood obesity and all the diseases that come with it are on the rise. I wish I could say that growing old is the only problem we face when it comes to losing weight, but we are fostering unhealthy patterns in the lives of our kids, setting them up to be one more generation plagued by disease and preventable hardship even in their youth.

We know the solutions though, don't we? Chapter by chapter here in this book, we are learning to exchange unhealthy patterns with God-honoring habits. Eating a healthy diet, getting quality sleep, staying hydrated, fostering healthy relationships, and keeping physically active are all cornerstones of a life well lived. The question is, what is stopping you? Are you living in the moment—or just surviving? Like those preschoolers at my son's graduation ceremony, are we looking to the future, full of hope, ready to make the most of life? Perhaps your ballerina days are over, but don't underestimate the swift impact of a few healthy changes in your lifestyle. We are not victims of the passage of time. Adulthood doesn't need to rob us of our dreams if we are healthy enough to pursue them.

Let's Pray

Dear Lord, every day You give is a gift. My desire is to live to an old age and to feel vibrant and strong. I know Your desire is for me to grow spiritually mature in the process. Lord, renew my mind. Strengthen my body. Use me for all my days for all Your glory. In Jesus' name, amen!

ten

When You Want to Be a Couch Potato

Over the last four years, I have had thousands of conversations with men, women, and teenagers about their health and physical activity. I can almost repeat in my sleep what the majority of them tell me. The kids go to bed, the dog gets fed, and then it's time to hit the couch and watch TV. Time on the couch *is time well earned*. I craved that time on the couch myself, and relished it each day. The couch potato pattern is persistent. Many of us don't get our rears in gear until the weight gain and lethargy lead to an unacceptable level of discomfort.

That was me. Drained of energy by two o'clock each afternoon, I didn't feel motivated to change. Dr. Bill Crawford, PhD, once said, "The problem with lethargy is that doing nothing validates the fear that nothing can be done." **It's a vicious cycle of triggers. We are inactive, so we feel lethargic, and because we feel lethargic, we become inactive.** Being a couch potato can rob us of quality time with our kids or getting outside to relish the beauty of the world around us. It can also rob us of our health and the enjoyment of truly living our best life.

If you have read some of my other books, you know I'm an advocate for rest and restoration. That's one thing. But being a habitual couch potato is another. A recent study showed that 86 percent of Americans spend much of their day seated.[1] Most are sedentary for over nine hours on average, and up to fifteen hours of their day is spent physically inactive. Yet the benefits of moving our bodies are well established. Improved mood, creativity, attention span, and performance are four big benefits. A habit of healthy movement lowers cholesterol and blood pressure as well as combats risks of cardiovascular disease, diabetes, and stroke. If that's not enough reason to hit the elliptical machine while watching your favorite episode of *When Calls the Heart* or a Clemson football game, I don't know what is.

Even though I knew I needed to be more active, I still found it hard to put it into practice. If you feel that way, you receive no judgment from me. I've been there! **Spiritually, I knew I needed a different kind of rest for my body. Lethargy is not rest. It is lethal.** The unhealthy pattern of getting off my feet was camouflaged as rest, even though I knew Matthew 11:28–30 (ESV) by heart:

> "Come to me, all who labor and are heavy laden, and I will give you rest. Take my yoke upon you, and learn from me, for I am gentle and lowly in heart, and you will find rest for your souls. For my yoke is easy, and my burden is light."

The paradox of physical activity is that the more active we are, the more rested and stress-free we feel. It's a euphoric feeling of "healthy tired" and satisfaction at the same time. We can thank God's design of our hormones for that. When we are exercising, our bodies release "feel good" endorphins. I don't know about you, but I need as much "feel good" as I can get! Science and major health guidelines around the world advocate for at least thirty minutes a day of exercise and strength training to maintain proper health. God's Word instructs us that true inner rest is found in Him—in taking our cares and concerns straight to God. This might sound a little odd, but I decided to put this challenge to the test and combine my physical activity with time with God.

My favorite means of raising my heart rate was a good twenty to thirty minutes on the trampoline with my kids, blasting Christian music. **Workouts plus worship are a winning combination!** During the difficulty of planks, I got into the habit of repeating Matthew 11:28 or some other Bible verse I wanted to memorize as a way to take my mind off the burn.

I began to transform. Not just in body, but in spirit. My clean eating lifestyle—in which I avoided eating processed foods as much as possible and focused on choosing more whole foods like green vegetables and lean proteins—removed the necessity to exercise for weight loss. When my mindset shifted in that way, exercise no longer became a chore or a "must do" to manage my calorie intake. As a result, I began to enjoy activities just for the fun of it. No longer did I feel the pressure to run five miles in the hills. Two goals I had for 2020 were to learn more Scripture and to increase my activity levels. Killing two birds with one stone eliminated my excuse that time would not allow me to fit both of those into my busy day. Quickly, I began to see that making those two habits a priority was God's way of answering my prayers for change in my life. He wasn't going to wave a magic wand and transform me, but He would show me that I could partner with Him to strengthen my faith and my body.

> Spiritually, I knew I needed a different kind of rest for my body. Lethargy is not rest.

This past Christmas, I saw a tearjerker of a commercial for the European pharmaceutical company DocMorris. It opens with an elderly man, living alone, reminiscing over family photographs on his wall. The next day, we see him dusting off an old kettlebell weight in his cluttered garage, and then every morning we see him struggle to lift it as his nosy neighbors look on with curiosity and disdain. The montage continues until Christmas Eve, when he joins his family for the holiday. Offering a beautifully wrapped package to his granddaughter, she opens it with delight, discovering a beautiful golden star within its folds. In the final scene, Grandpa raises her up to place the star on the top of the Christmas tree, and we discover why he was so determined to lift the cumbersome weight day by day.[2]

Like that grandfather, my new God-honoring habit began with one decision. That decision led to a week of fifteen minutes of physical activity per day. Slowly, I increased my minutes up to thirty per day. Simple. Doable. Life-changing. I did not set out to do thirty push-ups on day one. I began with five, pushing against a wall. Then eight. Then ten. Little by little, breathing out a prayer or a word of affirmation, or even letting tearful prayers flow on a solitary hike in the hills around my home, **I began to see my desire for more time off the couch and more time with Jesus grow from a decision to a devotion.** Devotion to my health. Devotion to God. I did not need to compartmentalize the two. Instead, I learned that they could complement each other. After all, exercise was a spiritual act of obedience, stewarding my body as God asked me to do.

For others, the frustration with weight loss comes because they are highly active but the pounds don't budge. So why bother? The lure of the couch is especially appealing when we don't see the fruit of our labor. The discouragement of working hard vs. the minimal payoff messes with our minds and, soon enough, we quit.

Jenna was more than frustrated with her weight loss. For years, she ate like a bird and hiked many miles every day. A cancer survivor, she felt like the medications she was on were simply blocking her efforts. Jenna hired nutritionists, tried every method that was popular at the time, and still had little progress. When she came to my husband and me for help, we sympathized. We also knew we could set her up for success. Skeptical, she tried our plan as a last resort. We coached her to hydrate, get good sleep, and eat small, clean meals every two to three hours. Intense exercise was shelved for the first week as her metabolism and blood-sugar levels stabilized. Then she slowly began to increase her physical activity. During her first week, she lost twelve pounds. That's far more than typical for a first week, and her weight loss stabilized to the recommended amount of one to two pounds a week. Her medically designed food plan ensured she was staying healthy, even though she was burning fat rapidly at the onset. She shared this testimony on her Facebook page:

> Hello, friends and family! I'm one week into my health journey and I'm down 12 pounds. I am literally stunned. I know many of you have seen me kickboxing, jogging on the treadmill, swimming, walking the hills, and eating clean and minimally for weeks on end with no change in my weight or appearance. With the three surgeries and the new breast cancer meds, I saw the scale just rising every few days, and I was in a panic. I worked with a nutritionist and an endocrinologist, and there was no improvement. I couldn't recognize my body and wondered how can it be healthy to be at this weight? I was demoralized but knew I couldn't give up. There was no chance that the oncologist was going to let me go off this medicine, so I had to keep searching for a solution. In the midst of my cancer treatment, my daughter said she saw this quote and thought of me: "She stood in the storm, and when the wind did not blow her away, she adjusted her sails." I needed to adjust my sails again. I had to try something new, and it is working! I feel good, have great energy, my clothes are fitting better, and I'm learning new habits. I CANNOT wait to see what happens next!! Thank you, Amber and Guy, for sharing this with me!

Two months later, thirty pounds were released from her body. She couldn't believe it, but she is living it. For Jenna, her unhealthy pattern seemed healthy. How could working out not produce results? How did exchanging that pattern for a God-honoring habit of moderation and regulating her diet with her physical activity make such a difference? Without enough nutrition and a good balance of carbs, protein, and healthy fat fueling her body, it held on to fat instead of releasing it. Once we got the combination in balance, her body was able to release the fat stores and properly regulate her metabolism. It wasn't hard. It was science.

God tells us that training our bodies has value. Developing our character biblically is even more valuable:

> For while bodily training is of some value, godliness is of value in every way, as it holds promise for the present life and also for the life to come.
>
> 1 Timothy 4:8 ESV

I'm more and more convicted that I can't waste my life. If I'm not physically well, I will be limited in what I can accomplish and how effective I will be for the kingdom. The two are not separate. That truth motivates me! I know that some health issues are out of our hands, but as long as it is in my power to help myself, I feel the need to do what I can.

The more I grow in my relationship with God, the more I see that He longs for us to live a life of abundance and influence. Our world is not home. That's what heaven is for. But as long as God gives us the gift of a new day, let's make the most of it. Even in this moment as you read, wiggle your toes. Do one knee lift. Stretch your arms wide. Slowly roll your neck from side to side. Do you sense a difference in your body, even in those small gestures? **Exercise and simple basic movements throughout your day don't need to be extreme, but they do have an extreme impact on your health.** Moving our bodies regularly reminds us that we are alive, and to live is Christ!

You may not be motivated by lifting your grandchild to place a Christmas star on your tree, but perhaps lifting praise and thanksgiving as part of your routine will impact your life in ways you never imagined. I know the couch has its appeal, but let me appeal to you to prioritize physical activity and spiritual rest for your soul. **Let's master unhealthy patterns so that we may honor our Master.**

Let's Pray

Lord, You are a God of strength and purpose. I don't want to waste my life or my abilities. Please show me how to be consistent in my exercise routine, and help me not to be lazy. Lord, give me victory, one kettlebell lift, one lap, one flight of stairs at a time. Let this time be an act of worship unto You. In Jesus' name, amen!

eleven

When You Travel

The flight attendant's voice startles as the airplane taxis down the runway. The usual standard instructions for safety are presented as a few passengers tune in. Most continue to read books or busy themselves on laptops before they are asked to stow them away. Soon enough, the crew announces that the beverage and snack service will begin shortly. And so, your vacation's food triggers begin.

Americans spend more money on food during vacations and business travel than any other expense, except for international travel fares. Hundreds of billions of dollars are spent on food services for travelers annually.[1] Part of the fun of travel is eating out, finding the best hole-in-the-wall in Philadelphia for a cheesesteak sandwich or feasting on Dungeness crab along the chilly coast of Seattle's famous harbors. But for those of us who want to stay healthy, we don't have to feel deprived when we eat out or go on a much-needed family vacation.

Mary was referred to me as a client by a mutual friend who had success getting healthy. On our first phone call, she was honest with me. "I'm not sure how I can do this and still enjoy a New Year's Eve trip to Las Vegas I have planned in a few months." She isn't alone in this concern. There's always a disrupter looming in the distance, waiting to trigger us toward unhealthy patterns. I honestly believe most people I work with are not looking for an out or an excuse when they raise the concern about travel plans; I believe they really do want to know how to navigate their health journey with real life!

The average American eats out 5.9 times per week! Even though cooking shows make up a significant slate of reality TV, only 10 percent of Americans actually love to cook. Even though it's five times more expensive on average to eat out than to cook from scratch, we are a culture committed to dining out.[2] We already know from chapter 5 that oversized portions while eating out can wreak havoc on our waistlines, so marrying our desires to eat out and stay healthy requires a balanced mindset.

As Christ-followers, we are not victims of our circumstances or our recreational choices. God wants us to enjoy time off from the grind and experience the beauty of our world. But everything we do in life is meant to be mindful and purpose-filled. Even planning how to vacation and fit DoorDash into our busy lives! Paul writes,

> When I was living among you, you lived in responsive obedience. Now that I'm separated from you, keep it up. Better yet, redouble your efforts. Be energetic in your life of salvation, reverent and sensitive before God. That energy is *God's* energy, an energy deep within you, God himself willing and working at what will give him the most pleasure.
>
> Philippians 2:12–13 THE MESSAGE

Being "sensitive before God" is a way of being mindful about all our actions, whether at home or play. Our energies, our focus for a healthy lifestyle, do not enslave us. We get to think carefully about the choices we make and how they impact our health. Our everyday moments become acts of worship as we obey God one healthy habit at a time. We benefit from both a healthy lifestyle on the road and peace of mind that we are overcoming old patterns. **Saying no to decadence at every meal does not restrict us, it frees us.**

As a mom with four kids, vacation for me means a vacation from cooking. When I began my own health journey, I had three business trips within the first ten weeks of changing my habits. If I was going to reach my goals, I knew that for me, just as it would be for Mary, there were two key things I needed to do in order to be successful. For any of us who travel for work or pleasure, being prepared and making conscientious choices will be the difference between weight gain and weight "release" from our bodies by the time we reach home.

> Saying no to decadence at every meal does not restrict us, it frees us.

In the days leading up to travel, preparing for how you will stay on your health plan will set you up for success. Preparing ahead of time protects your *why*. **As I made travel plans, the smaller goals for enjoying my trip had to complement my future goals of who I was committed to becoming—a healthier woman.**

Strategy will be a welcome travel companion. Try these suggestions:

1. Book flights so that you are already in the air during a mealtime. Airports are beacons of buffets tempting us by their accessibility to poor choices. Being airborne eliminates rushing through a quick fast-food restaurant on the run or being overly hungry because it's a mealtime and you are still waiting to board your plane.

2. Pack three or four meal-replacement bars or shakes that contain enough vitamins and balanced carbs and proteins for each day you are traveling. This way, you always have a healthy option at your fingertips for the airplane or while

bumping along a jungle trail—or even sitting poolside while your kids splash in the water. No need to be stuck with what a remote location or the swim-up bar has to offer.

3. When you arrive at your destination, make a quick stop to grab a pack of water bottles, or bring your own reusable bottle so that choosing water is an easy option. My kids don't even bother asking us for Pepsi or Coke when we are on the run anymore. They know I will simply hand them a water bottle!

4. Set your timer on your phone to go off every three hours to remind you to eat a healthy snack. Choose fruits, nuts, vegetables, and lean proteins whenever possible. Or those bars or shakes you prepacked in your bag!

5. Pick one meal a day to be your splurge, but keep it even-keeled. If you decide to enjoy the beignets in New Orleans, be sure to slowly savor the taste, and stop when you feel satisfied, not full. Having one meal a day that is not on your health plan is one thing. Eating three meals a day that are not on your plan will leave you feeling sick and tired—and probably emotionally drained too. It's not worth it.

It makes sense that planning will help you succeed when you travel or are eating out on a regular basis, but making conscious choices is the other way to battle the bulge when someone else is cooking for you. Preparing in advance, like we outlined above, is a conscious habit that won't just change the scale—it will change your life. Guy will tell you that one of the startling things about his health journey was how often he automatically grazed from our kids' plates or licked a knife laden with peanut butter after making them a snack. It's human to do so. But as humans, we don't have to operate by rote. We have brilliant thinking minds and brains designed by God to overcome patterns that do not serve us. When we realize that nothing in life has to be assumed, we open ourselves up to all manner of possibilities that move beyond our health journey. We begin to get an inkling that God is truly able "to do immeasurably more than all we ask or imagine" (Ephesians 3:20). Finally, we partner with God to be the dominant force in our life—not unhealthy patterns or robotic impulses.

One of my favorite writers and speakers on this topic is my mentor Dr. Wayne Scott Andersen, *New York Times* bestselling author and the tenth physician in the world to be board-certified in critical care. Dr. A, as we affectionately call him, says, "Most people are sleepwalking through their days, unaware and not conscious of what's happening around them. They are not sensitive to the reactive state they live in and how they are responding daily to the people, places, and things in their lives. They do not know how to treat themselves." Dr. Andersen suggests that the key to breaking this vicious cycle is to "Stop. Challenge. Choose."[3]

Let's say you are camping by a lake with your friends, enjoying the campfire and watching shooting stars. You have made healthy choices throughout the day and recently finished a fish dinner, roasted over the open flames. Suddenly, your friends offer you a skewer with an enormous marshmallow and a plate laden with graham crackers and chocolate. In the past, you may have thought nothing of it. You make quick work of browning your marshmallow before squeezing it between layers of cracker and chocolate and sinking your teeth into it. But now, things are different. You are not the same person. You **stop** before you roast the marshmallow. You think about it first, **challenging** why you might or might not want to indulge. It's helpful to take some deep breaths in this moment so you are mindful of your decision. And then you **choose**:

I've hiked a lot today and eaten healthily. I can have half a s'more and feel satisfied, you think. You take a delicious bite, knowingly, and then continue right back on your plan the next morning.

Or,

This looks wonderful, but I'm feeling content right now and proud of my progress today. I think I'll skip it this time, you affirm, and then continue on the plan as usual.

Neither scenario is wrong. Both are conscious choices. For those of you who have grown with me in turning from reactionary parenting, or arguing with your spouses, you know that triggers do not need to keep us living in a place of victimization. Our triggers—all of them—are opportunities. We can apply them to our emotions and our eating habits. When we stop, challenge, and choose, our personal and spiritual growth leads to the kinds of relationships with ourselves and others that we long for and have previously believed were out of our grasp. Let's not take a vacation from being mindful. Being mindful will ensure that the things we long for a vacation to provide—rest, pleasure, and wonder—will be found in the journey.

Recently, Mary and I met for a three-month celebration video meeting to discuss her ongoing health journey. She had just returned from her trip to Las Vegas. "I stayed mostly on plan, and it was easy," she said. "I had my champagne on New Year's Eve and enjoyed reasonable splurges, but I didn't go overboard." We both shrugged at the simplicity of it all. She was able to enjoy her vacation and revel in the ball drop at midnight without throwing all caution to the wind. It wasn't hard. Just intentional. Habitual. And on that call, we celebrated her then fifty-pound release of excess pounds she had been carrying just four months earlier. Back to reality for Mary did not mean feeling the drudgery of yet another vacation where she felt out of control and lived to regret it. She planned ahead, made conscious choices, and is the better for it in every way.

There's a well-known saying that it's not the destination, it's the journey—but your health journey doesn't need to end when you reach your destination. Eating out and traveling should enhance your life, not rob you of hard-earned goals. It's up to you. What do you really want? Put a plan in place, be intentional in your choices, and in the end, you will be able to take a permanent vacation from the cycle that is robbing you of your health.

Let's Pray

God, thank You for this opportunity to travel. This is a real-life moment, and I don't want my food triggers to ruin my opportunity to enjoy this much-needed break. You want me to be a mindful person whose actions reflect my faith in You and my choice to get healthy. Give me wisdom as I plan ahead, and help me to stop, challenge, and choose. In Jesus' name, amen!

twelve

When Losing Weight Is Easy for Everyone but You

Steve Jobs is a household name. You might even be reading this book on an Apple device, the brainchild of Jobs's genius. He famously once said, "Your time is limited, so don't waste it living someone else's life."[1] I shudder to think of the countless times I compared my life—and my health journey—to someone else's. Maybe you have too? Your third cousin once removed eats cake for breakfast and still doesn't gain weight. Last year, your husband and you got on the same health plan and he lost twice as much as you did. That medication you had to be on for six months brought an unwelcome thirty pounds, and there wasn't much you could do about it. These situations become triggers as we compare ourselves to others or are faced with extenuating circumstances. It doesn't feel fair! Comparison crushes our spirits when it seems that losing weight is easy for everyone but us.

The feeling that you alone struggle with your weight is isolating. Isolation leads to frustration, depression, and loss of hope.

Is that how you feel today? Is the struggle to get healthy a plague that hangs over you? Perhaps you have tried lots of methods to burn fat, but there it is, settled like cement around your middle. You look over to your right in your spin class and all you see is row upon row of muscular men and svelte women. Same exercise, different results. Why are they looking fit while you just want to *throw a fit* at the injustice of it all?

One of my biggest joys in recent years is hearing the hope rise in my clients' voices after a month on a health plan that is finally giving them results. When they "try again" one more time, hope is like a distant shimmer on the horizon, and they are tempted to think it is yet another mirage. Soon enough, hope grows as results begin to materialize. The evidence of progress boosts their confidence—but if you have little to no change despite your efforts, it's hard to believe that the state you are currently in is not a life sentence.

Sometimes we get triggered by comparing ourselves to ourselves. We look at pictures of ourselves from the "good ol' days" and wistfully resign ourselves to our current reality. Janie, a reader of my books, messaged me on social media. She wanted to talk. Her doctor told her it would be impossible to lose weight, as she was battling several autoimmune diseases and had gained forty pounds while on medications. I could hear the desperation in her sweet Southern accent. I had faith she could regain her health, but all she could do was mourn the comparison of her life before illness with life after taking prescription after prescription.

I asked her to borrow my faith that her body could be transformed until she could see it with her own eyes. *She did.* We got her system into a quick detox and regulated her metabolism with small, healthy meals throughout the day. In three months she lost forty pounds. Previously, her swollen ankles had not allowed her to wear shoes, but now she can take her pick of high heels if she wants to. Imagine if she had not reached out and instead settled for comparing her life before disease to her current reality, believing she was stuck. It was a highlight when Janie called me after her one-year physical with that same doctor who told her she wouldn't be able to battle the weight gain from medications. He was astounded!

One of the greatest basketball players of all time is, arguably, Michael Jordan. With six championship wins under his belt with the Chicago Bulls, his ability to fly through the air to slam dunk on his opponents has led to a massive marketing brand. My own boys ask for Air Jordans every year when they need new athletic shoes. With all his success, Jordan faced challenges and even failure during his career, yet he never quit. "Failure," he says, "makes me work even harder."[2] It obviously paid off.

Whenever we face a failure or an obstacle, we have two choices to make. We can say, "That didn't work. I give up," or we can say, "That didn't work, but I'm making progress toward finding what will!" **Our mindset will lead us toward mistakes or mastery; surrender or success.** Take a moment right now to evaluate your health journey. How many times have you tried to get healthy? I admit, I have tried stupid things that never worked. In high school I tried sniffing aromatherapy pens. In college I joined the cross-country team but never changed my eating habits, thinking the hours of running would simply be enough. After the birth of my third son, I lived on bland cabbage soup for days on end. None of those attempts produced results—just resignation that I was stuck with extra pounds and the frustration that goes with them. From high school to college to my adult years, seeing my friends lose weight or bounce back after pregnancies while I frumped along feeling tired and stuck messed with my head.

> Our mindset will lead us toward mistakes or mastery; surrender or success.

I am still a work in progress, but one blessing of my health journey has been allowing the Holy Spirit to remind me that I am unique, and that includes my body. Unique *and* wonderful. Psalm 139:14 says, "I praise you because I am fearfully and wonderfully made; your works are wonderful, I know that full well." But do we? Do we know that all God does in designing our bodies is wonderful? Do we know it "full well"? Or do we wish we were someone else? A baller like Michael Jordan? A little bit taller? A little less soft around the middle? You will never hear me say it's okay to carry dangerous fat on our bodies, but accepting the way our unique bodies adjust on a health journey is critical for hope to grow.

When your cousin posts a picture of himself eating cake for breakfast and then the next slide shows his spindly legs in a family photo, it's tempting to want to throw a pie in his face. Resist the urge. Things aren't always as they seem. Just because someone is within a healthy weight range, does not mean they are actually healthy. A large portion of people in the United States have a healthy BMI but suffer from chronic preventable diseases due to poor nutrition. You simply can't eat chocolate cake every day and have optimal health. So let's be careful about what we envy. Or better yet, let's rid the green-eyed monster from our lives for good. It's hard to keep your eye on the prize when your eyes are on someone else's progress in the other lane!

A professional swimmer puts it this way: "If you are staring constantly at what the swimmer in the next lane is doing, you are ignoring the things you can do. The things you are good at." He adds, "When you catch yourself peering over into the other lane, or measuring yourself up against other swimmers, turn back to your process."[3] **Comparing yourself to others will often result in their success, not yours.**

Turn back to *your* process. Stay in *your* lane. Fad diets may not work for you. They won't work for most. Your husband will lose weight faster than you because he is designed with more lean muscle mass and carries testosterone that aids his metabolism differently than yours. Those medications your doctor swears will prevent you from losing weight are rarely the only inhibitor to your success. The waif look of cover models does not necessarily mean they are living their best lives. **No amount of wishful thinking will burn more calories.** Be open to trying again, learning from your mistakes, and having the hope that change is possible, because with God, all things are possible. Make small, habitual changes, like memorizing Psalm 139:14, so your mindset shifts when you begin to compare yourself to others. Take a social media fast for a month while you begin your new health journey so you can stay in your lane. Educate yourself on why your body may be responding differently to food than it used to.

But whatever you do, do not give in to the despair of comparison. Remember that God made you uniquely and wonderfully. As long as we have breath, we have the opportunity to fail in the right direction, moving toward progress. Keep swimming, and soon enough you will find that the only thing worth comparing is how much better you feel now than when you started your journey.

Let's Pray

Dear God, I know You made me uniquely, so comparing myself to others does little good. I want my eyes to be on You, not on others. Whenever I start to compare my journey with someone else's, let me be quick to thank You for mine. Lord, I trust You to honor my desire to get healthy and that You will lead me to success in my own way. In Jesus' name, amen!

thirteen

When You Need Support from Someone Else

After several months of trying to contact Carol but getting essentially crickets, she sent me a message in the new year, bravely telling me that she wanted to try again. She felt embarrassed and unsure, knowing she had started and stopped the plan so many times before. We hopped on a Zoom meeting and I asked her this question: "Carol, do you believe that you don't deserve to try again because you have not succeeded in the past?" She teared up. "Yes." "Okay," I said. "Here's the thing. I want you to know that the last time does not matter. Nor the time before. Only this time. *This time is the only time that matters.* This time will be your time to succeed."

On her week one celebration call, she couldn't believe what she saw on the scale. Carol lost over twelve pounds! Because she had a significant amount of weight to shed, her loss was greater than average. As we talked, I asked her what she would be able to do in four months if she lost the monthly average of the ten pounds we aim for on our health journey.

Her eyes widened. "I could leave my house," she murmured. I wasn't sure if I heard her correctly. "I don't go out because of my weight," she explained. My heart swelled with the thought of that first outing. "Carol!" I exclaimed. "Do you know why I'm excited about that? Not just for you, but for everyone you will see and talk to. You are one of the sweetest clients I have, and your community is missing out on you. You are going to bless so many people by being in their lives again." I began to see the light behind her eyes by the end of our conversation. She was catching the vision that her health journey wasn't just about her. It was going to influence others too!

Several days later she messaged me. "Amber, I'm so excited. Today is day ten! I have never made it past nine days on a health plan before. We celebrated this non-scale victory with pure delight. Over the next few weeks, the scale continued to move in the right direction. Carol continued her healthy habits, one day at a time, and each day she got closer and closer to her goal. Even on an anniversary trip, she made use of *stop, challenge, and choose,* staying on the plan and enjoying a special meal with her husband.

The world we live in is facing a health crisis. Many of us feel like Carol. We have tried so many things before that we lose the ability to believe that "this time" can be the time we change for good. Taking steps to help ensure our success is one way to make this time the last time we begin again. The one thing that was different for me—and for Carol—when we finally made true progress in our health was having a health coach. When Carol struggled, she did not struggle alone. I was there to help her refocus, remind her what she is capable of, and offer tips from my experience to assist her in her journey. My coach, Tammie, did the same for me. Now I'm simply paying it forward.

Studies show that having a health coach makes a dramatic difference in your ability to lose weight and keep it off.[1] Those who are in a community and have others cheering them on lose more weight and keep it off longer than those who do not. At one hospital, researchers found that after six months, "Those who worked with a professional health coach or a peer lost an average of more than 9 percent of their total body weight. . . . This number is significant in that this amount of weight loss has been shown to reduce the risk of numerous obesity-related diseases, such as diabetes and heart disease."[2, 3]

I know myself. Without accountability, I get a bit lazy. My hope fades. I lose the vision of who I am trying to become. My goals begin to get a little fuzzy. But when I shared my goal to lose sixty pounds with my health coach in 2018, I knew she was going to gently but firmly check in with me and help me stay on track. And she did! I met my goal in less than six months. I maintained that loss for a year, and then in 2020, during a time when many people gained weight due to the stress and isolation of the pandemic, I was able to lose another twenty pounds. There is no doubt in my mind that I would not have been successful without the support of my coaches and their willingness to monitor my progress. When I felt like it was too hard, they helped me remember my *why* and reminded me what the alternative was—a life of chronic pain, psoriasis, and discomfort. If I had been journeying alone, I would have struggled alone, and that is much harder to overcome.

One of the main reasons we struggle with food triggers is because of fear. We fear that we may not succeed, or that the plan we choose won't work for us. We fear another disappointment or what others may think of us as we try to change our habits. Listening to fear is never a good idea. We must learn to do things even if we start out afraid. Over and over in Scripture, God tells us not to fear, but to move to action. When Joshua was tasked with leading the Israelites into the Promised Land, God promised that He would never leave him or forsake him. God urged Joshua to "be strong and courageous" on his journey (Joshua 1:5–9). On our health journey, we have a constant companion in the Holy Spirit to guide us. God did not leave Joshua, and He will not abandon us either.

Proverbs 12:25 says, "Anxiety in a man's heart weighs him down, but a good word makes him glad" (ESV). A fearful heart is a weighty heart, and when we are trying to lose weight, we don't need the added burden, do we? And yet, it's a "good word" that often turns things around. A good word from our coach who reminds us how far we have already come can pave the way for our next steps. This is yet another reason to invite others along with us on our health journey. Our resolve may slip and fear may try to dissuade us, but the steady arm and encouraging word of friends and health coaches are a welcome support system. If we journey alone and struggle, then we also struggle alone. That is much harder to overcome. But if we struggle and are in a community, then others come alongside us and encourage us. When we huff and puff and lose our breath along the rugged path, they breathe life and peace back into our hearts. **Hiring a health coach is not a luxury. It may very well be a basic necessity to give you back your life.**

Most of our weight issues are nutrition based, but because healthy motion and exercise are critical for ultimate health, having a workout buddy is another great way to stay on target. My friend Julie lives a few miles from me, and every week we commit to one or two hikes in our neighborhood hills. Setting that appointment keeps me from backing out because I don't want to be a flaky friend! One article I read recently stated that "a study in the *Journal of Personality & Social Psychology* showed that people work harder at what they are doing when they are part of a group versus when they are alone."[4] Julie pushes me to do one more big hill, and I thank her for it! When I was doing weight training, hiring a personal trainer kept me from sinking into the couch for the evening. I put my money where my mouth was, and investing in my health financially made it more of a priority. I didn't want to throw that money down the drain by not showing up for my sessions!

Health coaches, friends, and personal trainers are not going to magically appear on our doorsteps. We will need to become proactive in our health journey to reach out and find those who will support us. But beyond the support and accountability, having friends and coaches journey with us becomes part of the fun. Who wants to celebrate alone? *I don't!* Sharing small and big victories with others is part of the joy of connection as human beings. It's a basic need to relate to one another. When Carol shared her victories with me, they felt like my own. I was thrilled for her. I didn't need to be the one accomplishing something to benefit from the feel-good rush of endorphins. Her success blessed me as much as it blessed her.

There will be moments when things won't come as easily for Carol, but I will be there for those moments too, just as Tammie was for me. Ecclesiastes 4:12 says, "Though one may be overpowered, two can defend themselves. A cord of three strands is not quickly broken." Each strand that is wound together in unity to make one rope multiplies its strength. I remember sailing with my family through the San Juan Islands off the coast of Washington for several weeks as a young girl. Sailors flung massive ropes from their boats to the dock to secure their enormous ships. It was hard to believe that something so simple as a rope of several braids was strong enough to steady an enormous vessel such as those. When we invite others into our lives to help us get healthy, we rely on their strength when we are weak. Helping me helped Tammie keep the eighty pounds off that she lost the year before I reached out to her for help. Helping Carol helped me lose those last twenty pounds I was looking to shed after reaching my initial goal. Each one of us is a strand in the braid, mutually benefitting from journeying together.

May I reiterate an idea here? **Your companions may complement your lifestyle, but some of them may complicate it.** Choose wisely when you are on a mission of growth. Set boundaries where you need to and protect your process. My friend and mentor, author Jamil Frazier, puts it this way:

It's hard to set boundaries, shut doors, and separate yourself from people with whom you have a history. But it's also extremely necessary. Just like drug addicts have to leave their neighborhoods, and alcoholics need to find a new way home from work that doesn't take them past the bar, sometimes you need to get away from toxic people and places.[5]

I get it. You are afraid, or hesitant, or reluctant, or just plain resigned to begin again. The future seems uncertain. You begin to think that maybe others have something you don't that allows them to be the ones to succeed while you remain stuck. The voice in our heads is not always friendly. Having a health coach or a friend to drown out the chatter is one of the best ways to ensure that "this time" is the time your unhealthy patterns remain a thing of the past.

Let's Pray

Dear Father, You designed us to carry one another's burdens. Getting healthy is one of my biggest and most long-standing troubles. Help me to reach out for help, Lord. Align me with those who will be my allies in this fight against my flesh. Thank You for making me see that I can help others as I journey too, and that being willing to share my journey is what will make this time sweeter. In Jesus' name, amen!

fourteen

When It's the Holidays

D uring World War I, December 24, 1914, became one of
the brightest moments in history though it played out in
the midst of a dark and gruesome battle. On the fields of
Belgium, the German, British, and French troops were shooting
at one another, attempting to snuff out the enemy. Then the unex-
pected happened. The story goes that in the German trenches, the
soldiers decorated trees and lit candles. As the night wore on, they
reportedly initiated a Christmas truce that led to singing carols,
including "Silent Night" and "The First Noel." Carried by frosty
winds from one side to the other, the soldiers' voices sang of Jesus'
holy birth. Eventually, soldiers from both sides of the battlefield
dared to set foot in no-man's-land, the space between the trenches,
to greet one another. They clasped hands, shared cigarettes, and
even exchanged gifts until they were summoned back to their posts,
ready to engage in the bloody mess of warfare once again.

The Christmas truce of 1914 highlighted many reasons we love
celebrations of all kinds—even in the worst of times. Festivities

like these are a chance to gather from near and far and to focus on peace, kindness, humanity, and divinity. They are occasions to enjoy the company of others and to see our surroundings in a different light. Holidays give us opportunities to be generous and to receive the goodwill of others.

On that Christmas Eve, more than a hundred years ago, only one telltale piece was missing from accounts of this miraculous Christmas celebration: a festive holiday buffet. And yet, they were none the worse for it.

One of the first things that come to mind when we think about holidays is food. Many of our holidays center around meals. These aren't just any meals, however. They are often symbols full of meaning and traditions. As such, we place a lot of importance on what we eat. The idea of rituals and legacies isn't only found in the foods themselves. Preparations begin days and weeks in advance, as we go through the motions of preparing signature dishes. As rich as the meaning is behind these special days, it's easy to get lost in the mundane meal planning. Personally, I spent most years obsessing over recipes and food preparations, and based on the social media posts of friends and family, I wasn't alone.

Earlier this year, I sat out on my porch under a canopy of trees to enjoy the heat of an August day. I opened my Facebook feed to a happy announcement from a friend. "It's pumpkin spice time!" she cheered. Fall had not begun to show her colors yet, but coffee-houses were already ushering us into autumn with their seasonal coffee flavors. A few posts further down and another friend was sharing his favorite recipe for apple pie. My Pinterest feed was no better. Board after board highlighted the Thanksgiving holiday— and nearly every one of them was focused on what we should eat!

Thanksgiving is synonymous with overeating as the turkey is brined and families prepare stuffing, mashed potatoes, green bean casseroles, and every kind of pie under the sun. At Christmas, families prepare cinnamon rolls and streusel-topped coffee cakes or homemade fudge. Entire parties center around exchanging

Christmas cookies. The main meal of ham, turkey, or prime rib is followed by chocolate yule logs or English trifle. We toast with champagne on New Year's Eve after yet another decadent meal. On Easter, we look forward to a ham dinner and candy-filled egg hunts. Mother's Day and Father's Day aren't complete without a buffet brunch with shrimp cocktail and mimosas or a barbecue with juicy burgers. And what's the Fourth of July without hot dogs, baked beans, and apple pie a la mode?

Talk about temptations. These kinds of feasts take lots of planning—and we relish every moment of putting them together and then indulging. But afterward, we groan from full stomachs and full minds—full of guilt! As Christ-followers, we are called to have self-control, not allowing anything to rule over us except our one true Master, Jesus. That includes our food triggers and temptations. Genesis 4:7 warns us,

> If you do what is right, will you not be accepted? But if you do not do what is right, sin is crouching at your door; it desires to have you, but you must rule over it.

There is another sobering warning found in Proverbs 23:20:

> Do not join those who drink too much wine or gorge themselves on meat.

And another fitting admonition in Proverbs 25:16:

> If you have found honey, eat only enough for you, lest you have your fill of it and vomit it. (ESV)

Spiritually, we let our guards down during special occasions, but we are always to be above reproach, seeking to do what is right, even if others make different choices from ours. Yes, your friends and relatives may overdo it, but you don't have to. Temptation doesn't hold power over you unless you listen to it. **Every temptation tells us a lie.** Take a look at some of these common deceptions surrounding holiday food triggers:

God doesn't mind if you are gluttonous for a day.

You deserve to indulge.

If you don't eat the things that someone is offering you, you are rude or will hurt their feelings, and you are responsible for their feelings.

This holiday won't be fun or enjoyable without that traditional dish.

If you say no to these foods, you will be missing out.

It's impossible to make healthy choices during the holidays.

God is not really good if He wants to restrict what we eat.

If you are going to enjoy this celebration, you should go all out and worry about the consequences later.

God takes every temptation, *every lie*, seriously. His commands for us are not restrictive. They are protective. It's His love for us that issues guidelines for godly living, and we can trust them because we trust Him.

C.S. Lewis describes this concept in his book *Mere Christianity*:

People often think of Christian morality as a kind of bargain in which God says, "If you keep a lot of rules I'll reward you, and if you don't I'll do the other thing." I do not think that is the best way of looking at it. I would much rather say that every time you make a choice you are turning the central part of you, the part of you that chooses, into something a little different from what it was before. And taking your life as a whole, with all your innumerable choices, all your life long you are slowly turning this central thing either into a heavenly creature or into a hellish creature: either into a creature that is in harmony with God, and with other creatures, and with itself, or else into one that is in a state of war and hatred with God, and with its fellow-creatures, and with itself. . . . Each of us at each moment is progressing to the one state or the other.[1]

Every choice we make, holidays or not, makes us into the sum of our parts. Each daily decision shapes us into people who are healthy physically, emotionally, and spiritually, *or not*.

All the focus on food has put us in a bad way. If we truly want to fight the food trigger temptations around holidays, our growth in fighting temptation isn't the only thing that needs transformation when we want to get healthy. It's our way of thinking about our overall health that needs transformation too. This includes what we focus on during the holidays.

This is where the mind shift must begin. Every temptation to focus on food, whether during holidays or any other day of the year, is a temptation to focus on the wrong thing. It diverts our attention away from the best qualities of celebrations, and it fosters harmful thinking about what we eat and why. During holidays, food is viewed as pleasure, memory-making, and honoring traditions. But what if we thought about food for what it really is? *Fuel. Medicine. A gift.*

When I finally decided to get healthy and shift my thinking away from food as something that had more meaning than God intended it to, or that every item that passed my lips must always taste good, give me pleasure, and be enjoyed with every bite, I was free to view food as God intended it. It still gave me pleasure and was enjoyable, but detoxing from addictive sugars and processed foods cleansed my palate so that I could enjoy healthier foods that not only were good to eat *but were good for me to eat* too. My first thought about going out to eat or attending a party or celebration was no longer what delicacies I could enjoy, but instead how I might enjoy the experience itself, the people I would be with, and the meaningfulness of gathering with others.

I had room to think more about the people I would gather with and ways in which I could be a blessing to others during the holidays. Thanksgiving *truly* became about counting my blessings. Christmas *truly* became about honoring Jesus' birthday, and Easter *truly* became a day of worship. Sure, those elements were there before, but not in the same way as when I stopped crowding them out by obsessing on all the food.

Still, special occasions are opportunities to keep traditions— even food ones—alive. That's a good thing! It's also okay to make lighter versions of foods we love. We can enjoy a turkey dinner and a small slice of pie, or make recipes that are sugar-free or include more nutritious ingredients. Simply because something has always been done "this way" doesn't mean it always has to be that way if it no longer serves us well. You have permission to let go of traditions—and recipes—that no longer support the healthier version of yourself that you are working toward.

So many of us decide to put off getting healthy during the fall and winter months simply because we want to indulge for a few meals during the holidays. In essence, we have 261 meals to eat from November 1 through January 31, and yet we decide to set aside healthy eating during this season because we want to indulge for only four or five of those meals on Thanksgiving, Christmas, and New Year's. When we lay it out like that, putting off eating healthily doesn't make a lot of sense. **Let's not *take a holiday* from our healthy eating habits simply because it's the holidays! Each meal can make a big difference in our health.** A few meals where you go off whatever nutritional plan you are on won't derail you from your overall lifestyle of eating healthily and taking care of your body.

For many years, my food triggers around Christmastime had to do with my emotions. Born the day after Christmas, I often felt forgotten and overlooked. It doesn't bother me much anymore, but growing up I battled disappointment every December. Sweet treats were my soothing agents for far too long. As much as we long to enjoy the spirit of various holidays, they can bring a lot of pressure and stress, which also leads to overeating. For many of us, the loss of loved ones brings new waves of grief. The grieving process intensifies when their absence is magnified. Our hearts hurt and food is an easy and readily available quick fix. Turning to food to comfort us is a real thing, but it never fills the void. The quick fix of food for soothing can never replace the irreplaceable and long-term loss of loved ones. Let's not even try. **We only hurt our bodies by trying to remove the hurt from our hearts with food.** That's God's place, not food's.

> Praise be to the God and Father of our Lord Jesus Christ, the Father of compassion and the God of all comfort, who comforts us in all our troubles.
>
> 2 Corinthians 1:3–4

I can't help but picture those soldiers on the battlefield on Christmas Eve during World War I in light of this verse. The message of Christmas is that the Prince of Peace was born to be the Savior of the world. Jesus was a perfect example of God's compassion on mankind. He came to comfort us in all our troubles—and as those men fought one another across the trenches, the only thing that could entreat them to lay their weapons down and step toward one another for a few stolen moments of peace and joy was this truth. Yes, each holiday has its own unique importance for why we celebrate, but let's never let something as simple as food steal the limelight.

> We only hurt our bodies by trying to remove the hurt from our hearts with food.

Getting healthy and facing holiday food triggers does not have to feel like a killjoy. The opposite is true. It's wonderful to cherish traditions, and it's natural to look forward to a piece of Aunt Chika's pecan pie, but learning to approach holidays and celebrations with a new mindset is not a problem if we remember that staying healthy is its own celebration of life every day of the year.

Let's Pray

Dear Lord, times of celebration and holidays are examples of good things You give, but I admit that I have allowed these occasions to be opportunities for temptation and even some sin in my life. I don't want to miss the bigger picture! Remind me what really matters—that it's not just the food I eat. Forgive me for putting too much importance on food and giving it more power than it deserves. Transform my thinking so that I learn to focus on the people and the meaningfulness behind times of celebration, instead of all the things to put in my mouth. I trust You to help me keep the main thing, the main thing. In Jesus' name, amen!

fifteen

When You Hit a Plateau

Nobody likes a plateau—that dreaded period in your health journey when the scale will not budge. Few challenges to getting healthy are more aggravating and discouraging. After all, you have been steadily losing weight and getting closer to your goals. Not much has changed, so when the scale stops, you begin to doubt yourself. The fear of not knowing what to do to get it going again is real—and discouraging! It's the kind of food trigger that makes you want to quit. Thankfully, there are some specific factors that often contribute to plateaus, and understanding them can get you back on track to losing weight and feeling great.

When we hit a plateau, we often question ourselves: *What am I doing wrong?* Sometimes it has nothing to do with what you are or are not doing. One reason you may find yourself stuck is because your metabolism has simply slowed down. When you lose weight, you inevitably lose muscle along with fat. The Mayo Clinic reports, "Muscle helps keep the rate at which you burn calories (metabolism) up. So as you lose weight, your metabolism declines, causing you to burn fewer calories than you did at your heavier weight."[1] That translates as hindered weight loss. Knowing this is actually empowering.

There is no need to panic when the scale stalls. You have two solutions: You can reduce the calories you are consuming, or increase your exercise—especially building muscle—or both! It's important to always consult a doctor so that you are eating a proper number of calories and increasing activity levels in a safe manner. Give your body time to adjust to the new you that has been emerging on your health journey. At some point, your body will get comfortable at a sweet spot in your weight and want to stay there, but knowing you are not powerless to make changes goes a long way in restoring your sanity.

Ecclesiastes 7:8 says, "Better is the end of a thing than its beginning, and the patient in spirit is better than the proud in spirit" (ESV). Take the time to reflect on how far you have already come when you reach a plateau, even if you are only a few months into your journey. **Keep the end in sight, knowing that where you started is not worth returning to.** If food triggers really are opportunities, then a plateau is an opportunity to be still for a minute, consider how your patterns have already changed, and refocus on the end game. Take full advantage of that!

It's also an excellent time to do what I call a "system check." Studies show that overwhelmingly, one reason most people plateau is because they begin to loosen their resolve and start to revert to some of their unhealthy patterns. We aren't always aware of the impact these seemingly insignificant choices make when we are in the weight-loss phase of our health journey. We tell ourselves that a bite here or a nibble there won't hurt. We reason that we are halfway to our goal already, so going back to a bowl of ice cream now and then doesn't seem like a big deal. And for some of us, we can make those choices and be back on track, but for others, these choices lead to a stall in weight loss. Don't let diet fatigue sabotage your journey. Hang in there!

Remember this is a lifestyle, so keep your *why* in mind as motivation to finish strong.

One of my clients, Leanne, was growing alarmed. It had been several weeks since she had stopped losing weight. Even though the scale was frustrating, Leanne was committed to the process because after four years on insulin, she was finally able to stop her injections. Still, she wanted to lose more weight. We hopped on a call, and slowly but surely we were able to pinpoint the problem. During our system check, we went over her food journal where she recorded her daily food intake. She had started using some sugar-free liquid sweeteners in her water and coffee every day. Lo and behold, they had a high carbohydrate count that was blocking her fat burn. Once she realized this was causing her plateau, the scale mercifully began to move in the right direction again. Sometimes, evaluating what we are eating and drinking is necessary to catch the culprit.

Human nature likes to dismiss all those little things we add into our diet, but the body is a calculator that keeps us honest. When I do a system check with my clients, I recommend going back to logging food and beverage intake in a journal or app on your phone. By writing down everything you eat in a twenty-four-hour period, logging your liquid and sleep amounts, and even jotting down how you are feeling emotionally and spiritually, patterns or slip-ups emerge. This can reveal areas where you are unknowingly sabotaging your health journey. Seeing it in black and white makes us accountable and gives us a clearer picture of reality.

Another area to check is hydration. Remember, your body needs a minimum of sixty-four ounces every day. What are you drinking besides water? How much caffeine are you consuming each day? Is there anything you are adding to your beverages that could be derailing you? If you have slowly begun to drink less, it may be time to start setting those water bottles around the house or workspace as a visual cue to remind you to meet your quota.

System checks are not complete without evaluating your sleep and stress levels. The two often compete. Are you getting a minimum of seven to eight hours of sleep every night? Has your stress level increased, and is that added anxiety keeping your mind from restful sleep? Recently, I found that my stress was mounting. A broken-down car, a health scare, and an increased workload were getting to me. As a result, I wasn't sleeping well, which left me drained.

Emotionally, I became less capable of handling stress. A vicious cycle! In times when we are restless, Romans 8:31 is a comfort: "What, then, shall we say in response to these things? If God is for us, who can be against us?" Take time out of your day to meditate on God's truth, even if only for a moment. Proverbs 3:24 says, "When you lie down, you will not be afraid; when you lie down, your sleep will be sweet." **When we are on a physical weight loss journey, let's remember that we are a prayer away from a metaphysical solution to all our food triggers.**

Remember this quote: "We are what we repeatedly do. Excellence, then, is not an act but a habit."[2] Mindfulness about our daily habits allows us to correct our course when we notice that anything we may be doing has changed, affecting our results on the scale. After all, it's been said that making excuses burns zero calories—as does being unaware of how our environment and things like lack of sleep or stress influence our health journey.

For those who have been staying true to your healthy eating habits and have been regularly exercising, yet still face a plateau, don't despair! There is help for you. It may be that you simply need to mix it up a bit. Routines are healthy and predictable, but when they stop serving us, it's time to think outside the box. Your muscles have memory and they become conditioned to the same old thing. They need variety! I love to walk the hills around my home, but when I wanted to get the scale really moving, I switched to strength-training routines. If running has you hitting a wall, try incorporating workouts that involve obstacle-course-style training or martial arts. Trade your yoga class for a few laps in the indoor pool once in a while. **Routines only serve us until they don't.** Don't assume that what was working will keep working. It's okay to experience seasons in your health journey. Your season of high intensity aerobics may very well have served its purpose, making room for something new and exciting to pursue. If you want something you've never had before, you have to be willing to do something you've never done. Plateaus are a perfect opportunity to see your journey from a new angle and expand your repertoire of experiences.

Over the course of my life, I have discovered that obstacles are often the way in which our resolve is tested. I want to pass the test. In all areas, I want God to see me as a woman who perseveres and trusts Him to see me through. Psalm 18:29 says, "With your help I can advance against a troop; with my God I can scale a wall." It's tempting to think of plateaus as problems—walls that are blocking us from advancing, when really, they are resting places where we can consider our ways, inviting the Holy Spirit to open our eyes and give us wisdom and strength to march onward and upward. Plateaus will mess with your head if you let them, but why give them that much power? After all, you have already come this far. The journey to the plateau has taught you that you can change, and so the plateau is yet another chance to transform.

Let's Pray

Dear Lord, I'm discouraged. I don't want to be, but I am. I have worked hard to lose weight, and now the scale won't move. Help me to have wisdom about what I need to change and the patience to accept the process of transformation. I want to honor You with my choices, even when I feel stuck. I praise You for how far I have already come, and I trust You to finish the good work You have started in me. In Jesus' name, amen!

sixteen

When You Eat Mindlessly

Robin is an amazing cook. She spends time searching for and personalizing amazing recipes, planning menus, and prepping meals for the week ahead. Her reputation precedes her, so an invitation to her home is rarely turned down. I happen to be quite lucky that she is my sister-in-law and I get to benefit from her skills regularly. This past year, she committed to losing weight and getting healthy. It was a conversation—in her kitchen—the year before that finally convinced her to follow her brother and me down the path to wellness. Pretty quickly, Robin discovered how her "taste tests" added up and impacted her weight. Logging her food intake increased her awareness of how often she was ingesting calories without even realizing it! She made mindful choices and lost fifty pounds. The pattern of licking a spoon or dipping bread into a sauce for a taste test is a common one, but like Robin, you can learn a few key healthy habits to keep the calorie climb at bay.

It's common that after a week on our health plan, we hear from parents of toddlers who tell us how often they had caught themselves taking nibbles of leftover dinosaur chicken nuggets or finishing off a crust from their child's peanut butter and jelly sandwich. The subconscious act of cleaning their kids' plates left a not-so-subconscious ring around their middle. They weren't even aware of how often they had been eating extra food throughout the day! (This is yet another reason why using a food journal like I mentioned in chapter 15 is so helpful.) Guy and I had the same experience. Bite after mindless bite, we finally realized our mouths were not trash bins waiting for every scrap that had been left on our kids' plates.

Not long ago I posted on social media a video of myself throwing half a leftover cake into my trash can after someone brought it to a party. People were not happy! "Why don't you give that to the homeless!" one upset man commented. "You could have given that to a neighbor!" another friend lamented. The problem is that the cake I was tossing was not *nutrition*. Why would I offer a high-carbohydrate cake full of refined sugar (proven to increase chances of obesity, which is proven to increase your risk for cancer) to a homeless person, who is likely suffering from nutritional deprivation? If I don't want to harm my health by eating cake, why would I consider offering that to my neighbor? I'm supposed to treat them as I would want to be treated—so after enjoying our small tastes, the cake went right where it belonged. It may have tasted great, but as far as nutrition goes, that cake was trash. Waste. **Waste is not good for your waist!** Or your heart, for that matter. The experience online grieved me as it revealed how addicted—how consumed—we are by food.

We have not only accepted, but embraced, an unhealthy world. We do not see dangerous foods for what they are. We aren't just mindlessly eating. We are a culture that has labeled all food as beneficial when nothing could be further from the truth.

One of the biggest areas of mindless eating comes with our pattern for snacking. Researchers say that 97 percent of us snack during the week.[1] This does not surprise me in the least. I'm that mom who wanted to have plenty of snacks around my house for hungry kids—and their hungry mama. This might be reasonable if we were choosing apples and low-fat yogurt, except that's not the norm. This snacking culture, which generally involves highly processed foods or snacks high in refined sugars, has grown in recent years. Shockingly, 81 percent of the added sugars in our diet come from foods consumed outside of mealtimes.[2] In fact, adults are consuming an average of 3,000 calories a day—far more than the Food and Drug Administration recommends—without being aware of it. Because we are no longer preparing healthy whole food meals, we are left with cravings and addictions that don't like to wait. They plead with us to be satiated, and we listen. The gas station mini mart, the movie theater popcorn stand, and the twenty-four rows in the middle of the grocery store lined with granola bars and cookies and muffins and chips all enable our unhealthy pattern of snacking on nutrient-weak foods. They make us believe that it is normal, acceptable, and good. But the medical industry is currently devoting over fifty billion dollars in medical costs each year to treat *preventable* diseases related to this epidemic.[3] Americans are living unaware of how our typically unhealthy snack choices are robbing us not only of our health, but of a stronger and healthier economy. Imagine if we took all that unnecessary spending on the medical industry and invested it in our kids' futures by improving our educational system!

I do not believe that the obesity wave in our country happened by accident. Nor do I believe it is not spiritual. First Peter 5:8 says, "Be alert and of sober mind. Your enemy the devil prowls around like a roaring lion looking for someone to devour." Why do we dismiss this warning when we grab a grocery store cart? It's not beneath him to join you in the food aisle. How is it that we move about our homes and offices casually snatching a donut here and a bag of M&Ms there? The food industry has much riding on the hope that you will do just that. Revenue from snacks alone was projected to be nearly 500 million dollars in 2021.[4] Their big business depends on our big butts! I know—it's sad but true.

I don't want to miss the gravity of this situation for us spiritually. We are not alert. We are not sober. The devil is prowling through the aisles of the supermarket while we shop. He is relentless. On a mission. Subtle. Deceitful. Do not believe that he won't use your everyday moments to devour you as you devour the very foods that could put your life and the lives of your family at risk. He wants nothing more than to shorten your life and make you and me miserable. If we are not healthy physically, we may not be healthy spiritually. **Don't let your snacks become traps.**

Several of my books focus on the topic of anger triggers. In *Marriage Triggers*, Guy and I talk about the difference between righteous anger and unrighteous anger. Unrighteous anger is usually personal and directed toward others. Righteous anger wells up when we become incited over real evil in the world, and our vengeful feelings are directed at our true enemy, Satan. I get righteously worked up when I think about the damage he has done to our health by making obesity acceptable and normal in our world. Slowly but surely he has worked his way into our habits, making them appear reasonable. Bite by bite, he normalizes nutrient-poor behaviors. Little by little he erodes our self-control and then burdens us with guilt and shame. Temptation by tasty temptation he questions our resolve and makes us believe that forbidden fruit won't hurt us. *Don't think about it. Just do it,* he taunts. *You don't want to miss out on that pleasure, do you?* That was his tactic in the garden of Eden, and because it works, he keeps at it.

Please hear my heart. I'm not angry with you. I'm angry that our enemy has been gaining ground in our lives with his deceptions. I'm right there with you. I was considered obese before I began my own journey. My directness is an attempt to snap us out of his hypnosis. If we don't see our unhealthy patterns, we can't exchange them for God-honoring habits.

Colossians 3:1–2 reminds us how spiritually empowering our hearts and minds are:

Since, then, you have been raised with Christ, set your hearts on things above, where Christ is, seated at the right hand of God. Set your minds on things above, not on earthly things.

God is reminding us of who we are and whose we are. It's like saying, "Hey! You aren't dead in sin anymore. Remember? As a Christ-follower, get your priorities straight!" God designed our minds to lead our actions. If we set our minds on earthly things— like our stomachs—we will allow earthly things to shape our lives. (And misshape our bodies!) This world will pass away. It has no real value, eternally. The creation is not higher than the Creator. Setting our hearts and minds on things above is God's command to us. We would do well to follow it.

The urban legend says that if you put a frog in a pot of boiling water, he will leap out, but if you put him in a pot of tepid water and slowly increase the temperature, you will soon have a poached frog on your hands. The frog doesn't realize he's being boiled to death until it's too late. The slow burn is a sinister one. Our mindless eating is like that pot of water, slowly but surely conditioning us to believe all is well when our very lives are being threatened. If we don't realize the danger percolating around us, maybe, just maybe, we won't be able to do anything about it before it's too late. But here you are, reading this book. Something within you recognized that your food triggers needed attention—not by giving in to them, but by combating them. **Transformation does not take place on the scale. It takes place in the mind.** Well done, dear reader!

As an author, I love to write stories, but every one of us holds a figurative pen in our hands, and every day we write another page in the story of our lives. Each time we exchange an unhealthy pattern for a God-honoring habit, we contribute to the grander eternal story of God's best in our lives. The story does not have to end with our victimization. Romans 16:20 says, "The God of peace will soon crush Satan under your feet. The grace of our Lord Jesus be with you." That future day when the final victory occurs is sweet to consider, but we can be victors today. God tells us that if we "resist the devil" he has to flee from us. The initial line of this verse says we must first submit ourselves to God (James 4:7). Submitting to God takes the form of practical actions that become God-honoring habits:

Clean out the pantry and remove trigger foods.

Buy a cookbook that provides healthy recipes.

Join a health plan focused on lifestyle changes.

Pray over your grocery list. Thank God for His good provisions.

Sign up for an exercise class at the local gym.

Keep a food log or journal.

Notice marketing strategies that lure you toward unhealthy patterns.

Mindfulness mitigates our food triggers. Obeying God by stewarding my body didn't just impact me, my family, and the economy, it opened my life up to manifold blessings. Blessings always follow obedience. I long for change in me and change in you. I know the good things that wait for us on the other side of this journey, and I believe that we can arrive there together. I think it's sad that so many of us struggle with our weight and we blame ourselves. It's not really our fault. We have had an incredible adversary and a greedy food industry deceiving us for an exceptionally long time. We've gotten used to swimming in boiling water. But not today, Satan.

> Transformation does not take place on the scale. It takes place in the mind.

Not today, big business. Today, we are awakening to reality and its impact on our spirituality. Today, we are more aware than ever, ready to reclaim our health, one conscious choice at a time.

Let's Pray

Dear God, I'm aware that I have been mindlessly eating and that I need to become alert and sober-minded. I know better and want to do better. God, help me fight this battle so that I can overcome this pattern in my life. Let Your Holy Spirit nudge me in the right direction and help me to make mindful selections at the grocery store, eating out, and in my home. Thank You for never condemning me but lovingly convicting me. In Jesus' name, amen!

seventeen

When Your Favorite Beverage Keeps Calling Your Name

In order to live, they risked death. The men crouched low behind the brittle brush of the African plains, waiting. Hours passed. Finally, an antelope appeared, walking tentatively toward the shallow pool of the nearby watering hole. One of the hunters took aim, but before he could release his expertly crafted arrow, the beast startled and leapt away. The reason why quickly became apparent. In the distance, moving at a pace of fifteen to twenty-five miles per hour, a thunderous herd of elephants was making its way to the life-giving watering hole—the distance between this threatening company of wild animals and the hunters closing swiftly. As I watched the scene play out from the safety of my couch and beyond the television screen, my heartbeat quickened. The hunters needed meat for their survival—the antelope and the elephant herd needed water for theirs.

I grew thirsty just watching the scene play out. Sitting in the comfort of my home, it was a short twenty steps to my kitchen. With the turn of a knob, water flowed effortlessly into my glass. No need to travel for miles or take my life into my hands in search of the quench. Water is essential for life—we all know this—but somewhere along the way, many of us had a mindset shift. We began to think of drinking as a means of pleasure, or as a tool to stay caffeinated, or a method to unwind. Orange juice, sweet tea, martinis, iced mochas, cherry cola, root beer floats, champagne. With all those thirst quenchers at our fingertips, why are we still so thirsty?

We may not think of ourselves as addicts, but some of us are slaves to our evening glass of red wine or morning Starbucks beverage brimming with sugar. We can eat all the right things, but we need to examine our beverages too.

There are spiritual implications when we try to quench our thirst with poor choices, and we will touch on that in just a moment, but first, knowing the benefits of proper hydration and water is helpful. In chapter 16, we learned the importance of mindfulness. **Mindfulness moves us toward mastering healthy habits.** When we know *why* it's good to do something, we are more likely *to do it*. Experts say that proper hydration helps with weight loss and joint lubrication, reduces tooth decay, delivers oxygen throughout the body, boosts skin health and beauty (fewer wrinkles? Sign me up!), cushions the brain and spinal cord, regulates body temperature, balances your digestive system to reduce constipation and heartburn, aids in preventing kidney stones, helps to maintain your blood pressure, boosts exercise performance, and allows your body to absorb nutrients and minerals.[1] That's an impressive list, is it not?

I know. It's hard to resist when fall comes around and pumpkin spice lattes call your name. It's easy to supersize your Mountain Dew in the drive-through. But what if we don't count the cost? What if we continue the patterns that actually parch us?

If you were to drink only one serving of a sugary drink every day (soda, lemonade, sports or energy drinks), you could gain up to five pounds each year. But it's not just weight gain that is a concern. Drinking these kinds of beverages regularly increases our risk of type 2 diabetes, heart disease, and other chronic diseases. Even more alarming, an increased risk of premature death is linked to higher consumption of sugary drinks.[2]

Whenever we substitute something pure, healthy, and good with something less than those things, we travel toward trouble. As a Christ-follower, I find that this theme runs throughout several areas in my life. What am I fixating on? What do I mindlessly do? What are my coping mechanisms for stress? For disappointment? For fear? Am I using wine or sweet tea to satisfy a need? And is it really satisfying at all, or just a temporary assuagement?

The prophet Jeremiah ushers a sobering description of the people he was in charge of leading. They were in the habit of being shortsighted. God describes them as having traded the one true living God for a poor substitute:

> "My people have done two evil things.
>> They turned away from me,
>> and they dug their own water cisterns.
> I am the source of living water;
>> those cisterns are broken and cannot hold water."
>
> Jeremiah 2:13 ERV

I read the prophet's words and wonder how the people could be so dense. And then I survey my own choices. God is ready at the waiting for me to cling to, and so often in my past, I turned to food and drink. A false god if there ever was one.

Few of us must traverse hill and valley to find a good drink. We need not hunt down the nearest well or watering hole. We don't have far to go to find a distraction from our troubles either. We'd rather not face our circumstances, feel the discomfort of emotional pain, or embrace the reality of life's hardships. Instead of being open to growing pains, we numb ourselves. It's the flip of a switch or the pull on a handle or the push of a button, and we have access to many a diversion. It's easy to find something to drink on every corner. Still, we thirst. **Learning to satisfy ourselves with Living Water instead of these poor substitutes is a matter of the heart, not the stomach. God is our oasis. The Source of living water.** Anything we use to mask or manage our emotions and sorrows will only leave us thirsting anew.

There is a connection between our spiritual growth and what we put in our mouths. Stewarding our bodies is a spiritual discipline, not just a physical one. If we know that the drinks we consume are harming us, but we continue anyway, we devalue ourselves. To be Christlike is to place great value on people. Few of us would consider purposefully harming others, but do we care that we may be harming ourselves by what refreshment we choose?

When I first began to drink more water, unsweetened iced tea, almond milk lattes, and other healthier beverages, I had to get comfortable with disruption. **If our routine is making us rotund, we need a new routine. We need a healthy disruption to eliminate the unhealthy distraction.** At the time I was writing my last book, *Marriage Triggers*, and homeschooling all four of my sons for the first time. I lived on coffee and sweet cream creamer. I could easily make it to 2 p.m. without ever having a drop of water pass my lips. I was not in the habit of hydrating my body.

One of the first things I did was get rid of the creamers and drinks that were triggers for me. If they weren't there for me to turn to, it made the battle easier to fight. The second thing I did was purchase a few appealing water bottles. One had a message written on it: "Keep going, you are almost there!" encouraging me to keep drinking my full allotment for the day. Another was insulated to keep my water icy cold over the course of twelve hours. Guy bought one in solid black so he could put stickers on it from places we have traveled, or other points of interest for him—like his favorite rugby team or surf gear brand.

First thing in the morning, I got into the healthy habit of filling those water bottles and placing them around the house or in my workspace. Every time I entered a room or got in the car, there was a water bottle inviting me to take a few sips. I disciplined myself to guzzle each time I laid eyes on a bottle. At first, I felt like I was going to float away, attempting to drink upwards of sixty-four ounces a day. But soon enough, my water bottles became an extension of my arm—a true habit of mine to carry it with me wherever I went, sipping happily throughout the day. I noticed a significant change in my skin almost immediately. For years, I battled psoriasis and dry skin. It was so bad that the psoriasis caused my scalp to scale over like the skin of a lizard, and I began to lose my hearing as it spread to my ears. By the third week of my new hydration habit, I noticed my symptoms receding. I'd suffered through the impact of my condition for many years, but within a few months, my psoriasis was healed.

I didn't know what I didn't know. Many of my health issues were being exacerbated by my lack of hydration, inflamed by the liquid sugar I gulped down. I had settled into living with a parched palate and dry lips. I hadn't even realized these were issues until I began to feel better.

I often feel this way about other areas of my life spiritually. I say I want my relationship with the Lord to be sweeter, stronger. And yet I walk around carrying my burdens, using caffeine to get me through the day when Jesus lovingly beckons me to cast my cares on Him because He cares for me. There's nothing wrong with having my morning cuppa, but when I become dependent on anything to help me manage my emotions or internal struggles that are outside of Christ, then I am digging my own broken cistern, lapping from a leaky vessel. A distraction from the Divine.

Getting healthy physically requires that we get healthy spiritually. What is it that is keeping you from putting the can down? Do you believe you are not strong enough to deny yourself the temporary fix? Are you afraid of what might rise to the surface if you no longer drown your emotions? Do you imagine that it will be too hard, and that failure is a fate worse than death? Let's not give our drinking habits more power or credit than they deserve. Instead, let's remember God's invitation:

> Let us then with confidence draw near to the throne of grace, that we may receive mercy and find grace to help in time of need.
>
> Hebrews 4:16 ESV

Each new day we will face challenges. Each challenge is an opportunity to draw near to the "throne of grace." When we do, we receive the very mercy and grace of almighty God "to help in time of need." Are we ready? Will we do so? Is there grace enough to flow in our hearts as the wine flows down the drain? Mercy enough when we walk down the beverage aisle at the store? Help when the caffeine headache pounds? God says there is. This struggle to purify our drinking habits is a chance to draw near to God and to experience that He is who He says He is. Animals get it. They understand the value of life-giving water. They risk life and limb to seek what their bodies need. Our human brains are far above animalistic capacity, but perhaps the antelope and the elephant can teach us a lesson or two. They value life so much that they are compelled to go to the watering hole. Might we value our lives too, forgoing that which compels us to cut our lives short and leave us spiritually parched.

Let's Pray

Lord, I thirst for You. I am tired of being chained to my unhealthy patterns. Free me! Satisfy my life with good things and help me to purify my drinking habits. I know You alone can quench my thirst. Thank You for loving me unconditionally. I come to You first when I feel sad or troubled. Comfort me and refresh me. In Jesus' name, amen!

Section 2

Internal Triggers

The triggers we discuss in this second section are some of the most common ways that our own internal issues hinder us from getting healthy. We will discuss food triggers like stress, emotional eating, loneliness, and boredom. These internal triggers don't have to rule our hearts and minds. We can combat them with the truth of God's Word and find healing and hope as we develop healthy habits.

eighteen

When You Are Stressed

It was a typical day, and that meant my to-do list had more to-dos than could be done. I thought it would be a good idea to give the boys a day of mostly independent work so I could get ahead on my lesson planning for the next several weeks. Organization is a thing for me, and on this day, I had each subject worksheet torn and sorted next to each of my sons' chairs for the day ahead. Textbooks, reading material, workbooks, and supplies all neatly placed in order and stacked so they could work independently through the day's lessons. As each boy took his seat around the enormous dining room table, handed down for generations, their faces were obscured by the piles of schoolwork in front of them. Just the sight of it was enough to send my oldest into hyperventilation.

"Mom, I can't do this!" Oliver wailed. Typically, my oldest son is cool, calm, and collected. Organized like his mother, he is a self-starter and accomplishes everything asked of him without my asking twice. The workload in front of him was the same workload he had been mastering every day for months, but looking at it all at once, it became an unachievable Mount Everest in his mind. Quickly, I took half the stack and put it in the other room. His body relaxed almost immediately. I reassured him that he didn't need to stress, that the work was the same as usual and that I would help him get to each thing one at a time.

It was a good lesson for all of us. I realized that focusing on the big picture made the smaller, achievable elements overwhelming. It was stressful! Stress is the body's response to the demands in our world. A recent study showed that an astronomical 94 percent of workers in the United States and in the United Kingdom reported feeling high levels of stress.[1] Another study showed that while to-do lists seem like a good idea, if they are connected to deadlines and are unreasonable in attainability, employees become less productive as opposed to reaching their goals.[2] This is exactly what played out in our schoolroom.

Unfortunately, we happened to be doing a cooking element to our lessons that same day and we chose to make chocolate chip cookies—a Lia family favorite. Usually, we have lots of extras to give to neighbors, but not that day. The boys polished them off in no time. It was not a coincidence. Stress-eating isn't just psychological; it's physiological too.

Physiologically, when stress levels rise, cortisol is released in our bodies. Medical researchers say that "initially, stress causes the appetite to decrease so that the body can deal with the situation. If the stress does not let up, another hormone called cortisol is released. Cortisol increases appetite and can cause someone to overeat."[3] When you reach for a brownie or a bowl of ice cream under stress, it's normal to do so because, while your appetite is actually suppressed under stress at first, cortisol eventually kicks in, and cortisol is responsible for increasing our appetites. That leads to overeating! High levels of stress, if not managed, can wreak havoc on our health. As a former English teacher, I favor literature over math, but even I know that adding food with the hope of reducing stress is bad math. Stress plus cortisol will add numbers to your scale, but that triggered trigonometry never solves anything!

The negative impact of stress is far-reaching. Headaches, sleep disturbances, sweaty palms, gastrointestinal problems, anxiety, feeling overwhelmed, forgetfulness, low energy, frequent illness, and a rapid heart rate are symptoms of stress, to name a few.[4] Life during and post COVID-19 has fostered new levels of stress that most people have never experienced before. It's no wonder that obesity rose during that year and a half. **For the believer, we are never at the mercy of stress when God's mercy is available to us.**

One of the most beautiful verses in the Bible is one I have clung to over the years when stress overwhelms my heart and mind.

> But blessed is the one who trusts in the LORD,
>   whose confidence is in him.
> They will be like a tree planted by the water
>   that sends out its roots by the stream.
> It does not fear when heat comes;
>   its leaves are always green.
> It has no worries in a year of drought
>   and never fails to bear fruit.
>
> Jeremiah 17:7–8

Can you picture it? That tree, even in seasons of drought, is able to flourish and do its job bearing fruit. It has no worries even though conditions for success are not optimal. The man or woman who "trusts in the Lord" and "whose confidence is in him" produces what they set their mind to. The person who thrives is the person who is rooted in Christ. Being rooted in Christ means that the central part of any to-do list should not merely prioritize what we hope to accomplish, but point us to Someone to trust in. Cortisol is no match for Christ!

We can put in place all the strategies in the world to manage stress, but the believer has a defense against the harmful impact of stress and the temptation to feed it. The Christ-follower is blessed to lean on God and believe He will calm our storms. **Jesus doesn't just calm storms that take shape in waves and winds; He can calm the storm of hormones, like cortisol cravings, too.**

When I started my health journey, stress mastered me. By the time I was two years into maintaining an eighty-pound release of fat, I was physically smaller but mentally grander. My stomach shrunk but my brain power increased. Here's what I mean. If we are going to combat cortisol and stop eating our stress, we need to replace unhealthy patterns with healthy habits. Food triggers give us the opportunity for personal development and to engage our thinking brain instead of our emotional one. We learn to put habits in place to help us instead of becoming victims of our circumstances. Author and Bible teacher Joyce Meyer says, "We can't ask [God] to deliver us from the problem that we keep feeding."[5] Pray but take responsibility to install the healthy habits we are exploring in this book.

When Oliver panicked over his school load, he said he couldn't do it. I did two things that helped him cope immediately: I removed the overwhelming "list" in front of him, and I affirmed what was actually possible for him. When you feel overwhelmed by your responsibilities, do quick work to minimize your to-do list to three to four main priorities. When you hear negative chatter begin in your head, silence it with what you know is true. As their mama, I can remind my sons to take one thing at a time, and that they are capable. As adults, we need to do the same thing for ourselves. Positive self-talk is not weird. It's weaponry against harmful patterns that rob us of our health.

Guy and I work from home as health coaches, authors, and producers. Zoom meetings, long hours at a computer, and sitting down for meetings with executives at studios are common practice for us. We do a lot of sitting! When two of our colleagues bought stand-up desks, we knew one was in our future too. Being physically active helps relieve stress. Standing instead of sitting helps manage some of that physical and mental fatigue. So do lunches on the move. We often grab a protein shake and take a walk around the neighborhood on our lunch breaks.

For my birthday this year, Guy surprised me with an Apple Watch. The Breathe feature reminds me to stop and take deep breaths over the course of a minute to oxygenate my blood and calm my heart. There are apps available that have similar features, or you can set a timer for every few hours to cue you when it's time to stop and meditate on an encouraging Bible verse or take a moment to simply do a few stretches in your office for a quick break in your day. Recently, a client of mine turned me on to an app that incorporates calming nature sounds with soothing guided devotionals.

Not long ago, we added a kitten to our brood. She makes us happy. One of the studios Guy and I worked with in the past had as many dogs in the office as employees. Stopping to pet your dog or cat or listen to your songbird does wonders for the spirit!

My boys are in the habit of listening to jazz music as they fall asleep at night. I know firsthand the influence music has in calming nerves and affecting our minds. In graduate school, I was working relentlessly teaching full time and going to school full time, simultaneously. Talk about stress! Interestingly, my thesis for my master's degree was based on the premise that listening to classical music is food for your brain and can aid in academic achievement, specifically memory retention. It turns out my thesis proved correct. I performed an experiment among my high school English classes over the course of a school year as part of my research. Half of the students listened to Vivaldi's *Four Seasons* every time they took tests. Half of them did not. None of them knew what I was up to. Guess which students outperformed the other? You probably guessed where this is going. The students who achieved higher averages on tests were those from the classes listening to Vivaldi quietly stream in the background.

The great preacher Charles Spurgeon said, "Our songs should exceed our sighs." Classical music is one thing, but another way to reduce stress is to overshadow the anxiety with praise and worship. The psalmist's turmoil is obvious in Psalm 42:5: "Why are you cast down, O my soul, and why are you in turmoil within me? Hope in God; for I shall again praise him, my salvation" (ESV). He recognized that the first defense against stress and anxiety was to praise God in song and to reflect on his salvation. His song exceeded his sighs, and it made all the difference.

As a young mom, I learned quickly that when everyone is out of sorts, grumpy, anxious, and stressed, sometimes you all just need to go to bed. Seriously. Take a nap. If stress is keeping you awake, don't feel bad about getting fifteen minutes of shuteye on your lunch break or napping when your kids nap. Or maybe it's necessary to get to bed earlier. I advocate for a minimum of seven hours of sleep each night. If you are not achieving optimal rest, the healthy habit of sleep will go far in regulating your moods.

Don't forget to do things every day that bring you joy. The simple act of being generous when you tip your server at dinner, or taking the scenic route home, or finally signing up for that photography workshop reminds us that there is more to life than our responsibilities. Life is beautiful, and allowing stress to rob us of the good things God wants us to enjoy and the good work He designed us to do is not living our best life.

I can always tell when one of my health coaching clients is under more stress than usual. They confess that their eating habits have strayed a bit, and then they begin to list the burdens and responsibilities they are facing, hoping for some understanding. And they get it. I was the queen of stress-eating. I'm quite sympathetic. You may have turned to this chapter at a burdensome time in your own life. Common factors that contribute to stress are things like a to-do list you can't seem to conquer, expectations from your spouse that feel unjust, a house that has become more of a burden than a blessing, receiving a promotion you aren't sure you are qualified for, an event you are planning, a speaking engagement to prepare for, or perhaps you have said yes to too many things. If you are like most of us, you probably have little downtime scheduled into your week, and the pace you are pushing through is bringing you to your breaking point.

Food does not manage your stress. You do. The Holy Spirit does. I bet you didn't need to be told that stress-eating is not solving your problems. In the past, my own unhealthy pattern for stress-eating involved getting my four kids down for the night, changing into my pajamas, and queuing up an episode of *The Crown* or *Blue Bloods* while Guy scooped me a generous bowl of chocolate brownie ice cream, or on some occasions, mocha almond fudge. The ice cream would feel wonderful for about fifteen minutes. And then the little bit of stress that was soothed returned with extra stress over my ice cream binge. I was actually worse off than when I started. When I reached the most I have ever weighed in my life, just a few years ago now, it corresponded with some of the most stressful times in my life. It was no coincidence.

If stress triggers you to eat, you aren't alone. When we eat because we are stressed, we turn food into something it was never intended to be. We hope it will function in a way it can't possibly function, and we seek momentary relief from a temporary source instead of lasting peace from an eternal Provider.

Exchange your stress for peace. In the Bible, we are told that if we want to love life and see good days, we must "seek peace and pursue it" (1 Peter 3:10–11). We don't find it at the bottom of a bottle or bag of chips. We seek peace by instilling the kinds of peacemaking strategies laid out here in this chapter. Which ones do you need to pursue today? You can love your life and see good days. Your habits will lead the way.

Let's Pray

Lord, You are my peace. I want to stop doing the things that create more stress in my life. Help me to get better sleep, cast my burdens on You, and use food as fuel, not something to drown my feelings. Keep my mind in perfect peace because it is fixed on You. Lord, I want to exchange my human stress for supernatural peace. Thank You for removing my anxiety. In Jesus' name, amen!

nineteen

When Negative Self-Talk Overwhelms You

I have said some pretty terrible things to myself in my lifetime—usually about my body or my failed attempts to get healthy. Every one of them was an affront to not only me, but to God. In my heart, I knew that He wouldn't want me saying those things, but my insecurities, shame, or fear crowded out both logic and truth. Sometimes, we can be our own worst enemy. And make no mistake, our true enemy, the devil, loves to whisper triggers in our ears, especially when we engage in negative self-talk.

As believers, "There is therefore now no condemnation for those who are in Christ Jesus" (Romans 8:1 ESV). No condemnation. Not for our sin, not for our health journey. **If God does not condemn us, why then should we condemn ourselves?** God made us in His image, so to degrade ourselves is to suggest that God didn't do a good work when He made us. Those are dangerous thoughts. Psalm 139 counters that kind of thinking. The psalmist writes, "Your works are wonderful, I know that full well" (v. 14) to describe the way God formed our bodies in our mothers' wombs.

The struggle is real, however. You know how it is. We start a sugar fast, and by day twelve we're making scones with lemon curd and whipped cream, and we've polished off three glasses of wine. We tell ourselves we are failures. Worthless. Unable to succeed. Weak. "She's better than I am," or "He's stronger than I am," or "I'll never be able to overcome my sugar addiction," or "My family culture won't let me eat healthily." We sink in shame or steam with anger toward ourselves when we do things we don't want to do.

My friend Vicki, a fellow health coach in my community group, told me about the time she made a chocolate cake for her husband. She took a slice before he got home from work and, before she could stop herself, one slice became two and then three. *One more slice is no big deal,* she thought. Half the cake was eaten in short order. She knew she couldn't present half a cake to her husband, so she reasoned with herself that it would be best to finish it off. Which she did. And then she quickly made a second cake before her husband made it home. "I told myself that I couldn't let anyone know I had eaten an entire cake!" she said. "I didn't want my husband to know that I lacked self-control." That was a turning point for her. Eventually, she confessed her tendency to overeat. Being honest with herself allowed her to be honest with her friends and family. Only when she stopped the negative self-talk was she able to make a decision to own her reality and begin the journey to healthier choices and God-honoring habits. She lost sixty-seven pounds and found freedom from the voice in her head that kept her living in a place of shame.

> If God does not condemn us, why then should we condemn ourselves?

The chatter in our minds is often unfriendly. Our coaching team calls it "Stanley chatter." Stanley's a bad dude. His MO is fear, lies, and discouragement. The chatter is statements like "My friends have faster metabolisms, and I am stuck with what I've got," or "I'm just big boned," or "Everyone in my family looks like this.

It's just my genes." We listen to Stanley and tell ourselves things like "I can't give up tortillas," or "It's too hard to exercise in cold weather," or "Tomorrow I will begin a diet, so today I may as well indulge." But tomorrow never comes. The things we think today are the same things we will think tomorrow if we don't disrupt our unhealthy pattern of thinking. *Stanley's got to go!*

The apostle Paul wrestled with his thought life too. "I don't really understand myself, for I want to do what is right, but I don't do it. Instead, I do what I hate" (Romans 7:15 NLT). It's one thing to know what is right or even to *do* what is right, but it's a completely different thing to *think* what is right. **Somewhere in between knowing what is right and doing what is right is the challenge to think what is right.** Whatever we think will have the greatest impact on our actions.

Second Corinthians 10:5 says,

> We demolish arguments and every pretension that sets itself up against the knowledge of God, and we take captive every thought to make it obedient to Christ.

I love the word *demolish* here. If you have ever seen a wrecking ball take down a building, you know the power behind a demolition team. **We need to take a holy wrecking ball to the thoughts and excuses and lies and fears that we play in our minds.** It's not too strong of language to suggest here that some of the arguments we have been making about obeying God in the area of food need to be wiped out and obliterated from our minds.

To take something "captive" means it does not have free rein. I think of this every time we take our boys to a zoo. Recently we went to San Diego and visited their world-famous zoo. We came around a bend to the lion habitat. A massive cat came right over to where we stood, stared me in the eye, and roared with such strength and volume that I shook in my flip-flops. I knew the glass formed a barrier between us, but it gave me little comfort. He and his impressive mane stood only ten feet from my face. I knew the lion would make short order of making me his lunch if we were on his natural turf, uninhibited by the barriers that kept him on one side and me on the other. Scientists say that a lion's roar may have the power to paralyze its prey. A lion's roar can be as loud as 114 decibels—about twenty-five times louder than a gas-powered lawn mower.[1] I understand that now. I wish all animals could roam free and unharmed in the wild, but it struck me that though this lion was captive, he still had his paralyzing roar. Its wild expanse could not be contained by glass.

Some of you are already making headway on your health journey, but even though you have made progress in your thinking patterns and are getting better at silencing the "chatter," there is still an echo chamber resounding in your ears of thoughts from your past. The negative self-talk is captive, but it still paces back and forth on occasion, trying to rattle your cage. When those times come, don't let them escape. They don't have the same power over you they used to have, but the lions of your thought life may still try to pierce you with their gaze and cause you to stumble with the rumble.

When that happens, Philippians 4:8 gives us a holy filter for our thought life:

> Finally, brothers and sisters, whatever is true, whatever is noble, whatever is right, whatever is pure, whatever is lovely, whatever is admirable—if anything is excellent or praiseworthy—think about such things.

Whenever we talk about habit formation, it begins with identifying the unhealthy pattern and then exchanging it for a God-honoring habit. But take it a step further. When it's negative self-talk, don't just exchange it. Demolish it. When the lie, excuse, or fear comes to mind, that's the moment of truth. Evaluate whether that thought is true. Ask yourself if it is lovely. Consider whether it is admirable. Is it right? Is it noble? If not, then it's time to strap on your seat belt, shift into gear, and swing that wrecking ball.

"I'm just big boned" is replaced with "I've never actually measured my bones. These rolls of fat have nothing to do with bone structure. This is excess fat and it's not good for me. It is possible to change that."

"I'm just weaker than she is. There is something wrong with me that makes me fail every time" is replaced with "I can do all things through Christ who strengthens me—even choosing the salad instead of the pasta."

"I can't lose weight because my doctor says this medication will cause me to gain, and there is nothing I can do about it," is replaced with "My girlfriend who is on the same medication as I am has been able to lose forty pounds, so maybe my doctor doesn't know everything and I should learn about her plan."

"It's too hard to get healthy when my husband and kids still eat junk," is replaced with "I make my own choices. Nobody is forcing me to eat brownies. I do the shopping and cooking, so they can learn to eat healthier too, or make things for themselves that they prefer. It doesn't mean I have to join them when they could join me."

"I'm hitting menopause, and this is just the way it is going to be," is replaced with "There are lots of menopausal women who are not obese. There must be more to the story than being ruled by hormones. I can research and find ways to keep my weight in check with my body's changing dynamics."

Learning to challenge our thoughts and make them obedient unto Christ isn't just a good tool for getting physically healthy. The renewing of our minds is also critical for every aspect of our lives. Your health journey is not just about burning fat but burning down every thought that blazes a wrong trail on your path to success. Jesus is our friend. Do the words you speak to yourself sound like something a friend would say? Or an enemy? The answer to that question and these practical ways of combating negative self-talk will help you face your food triggers and embrace the truth that you are valuable and loved beyond measure.

You are not stuck or paralyzed by your thoughts. Yes, your enemy is like a roaring lion seeking whom he may devour. But 2 Chronicles 16:9 says, "For the eyes of the LORD range throughout the earth to strengthen those whose hearts are fully committed to him." God is stronger than any mammal. The sound of His voice is more powerful than the voice of a lion—or Stanley—and certainly no match for the man or woman committed to acting on truth.

Let's Pray

Dear Lord, please silence the chatter in my head that tries to discourage me and lie to me. I don't want to listen to my own negative self-talk anymore. I invite Your goodness and grace to rule my mind as I exchange and demolish anything that is not true or good or praiseworthy. Thank You, Lord, for speaking truth to my heart and for loving me and accepting me. In Jesus' name, amen!

twenty

When You Are Lonely

Food makes a lousy friend.

During many seasons of my life, loneliness breathed down my neck, creeping into the quiet moments of my day. Feeling alone, even if we are surrounded by others, triggers many of us to fill the hole with food. The easy access and the traditions of comfort we associate with food make it a frequent choice for soothing the ache we feel. The problem is that the comfort lasts only as long as the food on the plate does, and that's simply not long enough to satisfy.

Psychologist Dr. Amy Sullivan explains that "loneliness isn't the same thing as social isolation. It's more about how you perceive your level of connectedness to others. . . . Someone who's socially isolated and doesn't have a lot of social contacts may not feel lonely at all, but someone else may feel lonely even when they're surrounded by lots of people."[1]

If you feel like snacking when you are lonely, there is a good reason for that. We can thank cortisol once again. Feeling left out or alone releases cortisol. We have already learned that cortisol triggers cravings to eat, so the lonelier we are, the more we may battle overeating.

While loneliness does not always equal boredom, that is the case for some of us. I remember when my kids went away to church camp for the first time. It was a happy day when I put them on the church bus. I knew they were going to have a lot of fun and be fed spiritually, but the happiness gave way to a strange void in my heart by dinnertime. I realized just how much of my day was parenting, cooking, and interacting with them.

By evening, I was at a loss to know what to do with myself. Making food seemed like a productive thing to do. I caught myself making far more food than Guy and I needed for dinner. The next day I found myself scanning the pantry for no particular reason. I had extra time on my hands, and because I did not plan for that void, I felt a little bored, a little depressed. Without something positive or productive to distract me, the kitchen lured me in. Thankfully, I caught myself before too much damage was done, and made plans that were far better for me than scouring my refrigerator.

My best friend, Joanne, is single and has no children at home. A former physical education teacher, she likes to keep fit and understands the value of eating clean and keeping active. Still, the long winters in Montana where she now lives can feel isolating.

Joanne and I are kindred spirits. We are both triggered by sugar. So when the loneliness kicks in, Joanne reaches out to her friends to go on a hike, plans a drive to her local hot springs, or works on a project for her online business. She makes her quiet time with God a priority, prepares a healthy breakfast, and fits in a thirty-minute aerobics video to get her heart pumping before the day begins. Is she still lonely at times? Sure. But Joanne is intentional to nurture God-honoring habits to combat those feelings and any urge to binge eat.

One of the things I love most about Joanne is that when she feels particularly isolated, she actively looks for ways to be a blessing to someone else. She writes notes or sends text messages to people God puts on her heart, offers her expertise in education by filling in for teachers when they need a substitute in her local school district, and tries to live in the moment of today instead of dwelling on a future that feels uncertain. She also knows that I am a phone call away when the snack attack hits her! Joanne is a great example of being disciplined, despite occasional loneliness.

At the times when I am the loneliest, I find I become the most undisciplined. My fellow health coach Jamil Frazier says, "Discipline is constantly choosing between what you want now and what you want most." It means learning to "give up the good things in the moment for great things in the future."[2] At this moment, are you lonely? Do cheddar herb biscuits drenched in butter sound good? Possibly. *But what sounds great?* Releasing your extra weight and feeling your best? Opening up to the healing of your heart by the Holy Spirit? Having long-term satisfaction instead of temporary enjoyment? I want to be the kind of woman who is quick to give up the good for the great! Do you?

For a long time, I found it difficult connecting with women, even when I wanted to, especially as a young mom in a new town. And then life got more complicated. For the last ten years I have not been the greatest friend. Deep in ministry and often overwhelmed with homeschooling and running a business, my priorities limit my availability to keep up friendships. I've chosen to mostly nurture them within my family circle and one or two childhood friends. I'm sure I have disappointed some people. Whenever that longing for friendship creeps in, I remind myself that I am never truly friendless.

Proverbs 18:24 says, "A man of many companions may come to ruin, but there is a friend who sticks closer than a brother" (ESV).

What a friend we have in Jesus! There is no greater love than when He laid down His life and called us His friends (John 15:13). It's hard to remain poor in spirit when we grasp the divine friendship we have with the Lord. **God always oversees; He never overlooks.** Lonely as we may feel, we are not forgotten.

I know we can be lonely in a crowd, but for those who have lost a loved one, the emptiness fills every waking moment. I remember when Guy and I miscarried twins two years after Oakley, our third son, was born. The pain I felt for them when they passed was like a continual punch in the gut. In the midst of my grief and loneliness, I felt the strong need to praise God in my pain. Days after the loss, I wrote,

Sometimes, the sacrifice of praise that we offer is nearly unspeakable. It's the quiet raging of a heart that knows unwaveringly that God is good when bad things happen. It's the silent tears that fall knowing without a doubt that God is capturing each one to hold in a bottle. It's the ability to minister to others walking a hard road when your own pain tempts you to say that you have nothing left to give. And it's the hope you have when all that you hoped for is gone. It's keeping your head above the waves of grief that keep coming. Sometimes, the sacrifice of praise is simply knowing that you don't have to understand.

When I look back, I realize that my weight gain increased dramatically after my miscarriage. I know that while I turned to God, I also turned to food. That doesn't make me a bad Christian. It makes me human. I hope that gives you some grace for yourself too.

At first the food was for comfort. As I boxed up the new infant clothes my babies would never wear or had to tell one more person about my loss, the pain would swell in my heart. **Instead of letting my difficult circumstance have its way in refining me, I used refined sugar to numb some of the sting.** Eventually it simply morphed into an unhealthy pattern. Three years later, our happy surprise, Quade, was born. It was after his birth that I knew I needed to stop using food for comfort and filling the gap between my heart and my hurt. Jesus needed to stand in the space between because only He could truly satisfy. The Swedish pancakes with lingon-berry butter simply weren't doing it. It sounds sacrilegious to even consider it, but when we are sad and lonely, we don't always think rightly. Yet again, Jesus covers even that, with His love and grace.

I wish I could give you a big hug right now. I know loneliness is hard. God knows too. He's familiar with all our sufferings. His compassion does not dim when the refrigerator light goes on in the middle of the night because we can't sleep and want to eat. Jesus stands beside us in the dark and tenderly beckons us to look to Him instead.

In 1 Timothy 5:5–6, the letter advises a widow "left all alone" and who is in need. Timothy instructs her to put her "hope in God" and to continue to pray for help "night and day." He goes on to say, "But the widow who lives for pleasure is dead even while she lives." Notice the difference. When we are lonely, alone, facing grief or loss, we can turn to prayer or pleasure. We can let the pain push us toward God or numb it with other things that will only prolong our suffering.

The God-honoring habit of turning Bible verses into prayers has blessed my life over the years. If loneliness is a food trigger for you, Psalm 25:16 (ESV) is a perfect passage to cry out to the Lord with:

Turn to me and be gracious to me, for I am lonely and afflicted.

Loneliness doesn't have to be a permanent condition. Take Timothy's advice and the psalmist's words and turn them into your own prayers. Put your hope in God. Offer the sacrifice of praise for your circumstances in spite of them. God created us for connection with Him. Let your loneliness lead you to His feet. **Your relationship with God is better than your relationship with food.** And the more connected you are in your relationship with God, the less lonely you'll feel. The less lonely you feel, the less likely you are to use food for comfort.

Like Joanne, let's put in place protections against loneliness, leaning on our friends in community, doing the good work God has set before us to do, and being disciplined in our habits toward healthy living. I don't know anyone who has never experienced a season of loneliness. It is part and parcel of our earthly experience.

Let me remind you of Romans 12:12: "Rejoice in hope, be patient in tribulation, be constant in prayer" (ESV). Do you feel a glimmer of hope that you can face your food triggers? That your loneliness will not last forever? Rejoice in that hope! The challenges and tribulations will still come. Dessert bars. Wine lists. Charcuterie boards laden with cheese and Parmesan crisps. Valentine's Day chocolates. Keep on keeping on, knowing that nothing is sweeter than the goodness of the Lord and His love for you. It's better to be alone in the desert and in the center of God's will than anywhere else, and yet He is only a prayer away from your lonely heart.

Let's Pray

Father, I'm lonely. My heart aches and I feel so alone. I turn to food for comfort, but it never solves my problem. I need You to change this pattern in my life. Lord, fill my heart with Your joy and happiness in due season. I want to be satisfied with You alone. Help me to make healthy choices when I feel lonely, that I may experience a closer relationship with You. In Jesus' name, amen!

twenty-one

When You Are
Addicted to Sugar

G uy had the kids out for a daddy day. The time was mine to write, get things done around the house, and maybe read a good book for a few stolen moments. I started out the morning feeling productive, but soon enough my mind began to wander and fixate on food. Before long, the image of strawberry shortcake layer cake from one of my favorite bakeries came to mind. Setting aside my laptop, I grabbed my coat and set off for the store.

Much to my dismay, the bakery was out of their strawberry shortcake layer cake. The nerve. But that didn't stop me. Another bakery was across town. Off I went. Sadly, that location was also short on shortcake. An hour and a half later, I had not done my writing, tidied the house, or read a good book. As I got back in my car, I considered heading to a third location, but mercifully, reason began to set in, and I turned toward home.

Why on earth would a grown woman with things to do waste her time hunting for cake? Because that's what sugar addiction does. I wonder, what lengths have you gone to for sugar? How many candy wrappers have you hidden? Or milkshake cups have you ditched before arriving home? Who has become a baker for the love of sharing but mostly for consuming? Me. That was me.

Author Yuval Noah Harari writes, "In 2012, about 56 million people died throughout the world; 620,000 of them died due to human violence (war killed 120,000 people, and crime killed another 500,000). In contrast, 800,000 committed suicide, and 1.5 million died of diabetes. Sugar is now more dangerous than gunpowder."[1] We have every right to be up in arms about all manner of addictions, and yet very few of us are alarmed about the sheer magnitude of sugar in our diets. Sugar isn't just sweet; it can be deadly. Our body's chemical response to sugar is comparable to that of potent drugs we would never willingly ingest or offer to our kids, but that day, its impact proved itself in my unhealthy patterns, driving all over town in search of a fix.

My crusade for cake was not because I lacked willpower. It was not because I was weak. Satan wants us to feel shame over our cravings, but in *Food Triggers*, we are learning that so much of this journey is physiological as well as spiritual. Researchers say that insulin rises in response to eating sugar and flour in refined food. That insulin then blocks leptin, which suppresses hunger.

In one study, mice were fed high-glycemic foods, and as insulin rose in their blood, the mice began eating continually and stopped moving. Mice are not known for their willpower. Or their spirituality. That had nothing to do with it. It's not because they were weak. It was because the refined foods flipped the metabolic switch.[2] This is why we binge on brownies after a long day or travel to the far end of the galaxy for a Milky Way bar. No wonder the average American eats about seventeen teaspoons of added sugar a day, roughly twice the amount recommended for men and three times the recommended amount for women.

The other factor is that sugar and flour feed our pleasure centers in our brains. Food manufacturers know this, and because they want us to buy more, they add sugar to many of the foods we routinely eat. Another study on rats showed that "Oreo cookies activate more neurons in the pleasure center of the rats' brains than cocaine does (and just like humans, the rats would eat the filling first)."[3] Our brain chemistry literally becomes altered by repeatedly ingesting these substances.

Dr. Wayne Scott Andersen, trained in open-heart surgery, says that if we continue to eat these sugar-saturated and refined foods, "the brain adapts rapidly and starts to thin out the dopamine receptors" in our brains. What happens next explains why the cravings rise within us. The receptors in our brains begin to "down-regulate, so now you lack the ability to feel the same level of pleasure unless you eat larger amounts to stimulate enough dopamine release."[4] It's a perfect storm of pleasure-seeking poison for mind and body. **Instead of starving our bodies of nutrition and nourishing our sugar cravings, let's starve the cravings and nourish our bodies.**

One practical thing I did when I cut back on processed foods and refined sugars was have a frank conversation with my family. I wanted them to support me in my journey. My children understood why I was not going to be bringing home cartons of ice cream or take them for donut runs on Saturday mornings anymore. They loved me and wanted their own bodies healthy too, so we all had a stake in my journey. Along with cleaning out trigger foods from my kitchen, we celebrated healthy choices we made during the day as a family.

The emphasis switched to all we were gaining, rather than what we were eliminating, and in so doing, overcoming this stronghold in my life became a blessing for my children and husband too.

By ridding our homes of addictive foods, we can't reach for them when we feel weak. They simply are not accessible. When I purged our pantry of my trigger foods, I was forced to engage my thinking brain to evaluate why I felt a craving. It also forced me to make a healthier choice. I would eat a serving of almonds or low-fat cottage cheese because those were my only options at the time, but they were good choices. Romans 13:14 (ESV) says,

> But put on the Lord Jesus Christ, and make no provision for the flesh, to gratify its desires.

Yes, we can still hop in the car to find a fix, but when we decide to be conscious about what we are eating, engage the support of family and friends, and detox our deep freezer, we no longer mindlessly allow temptation to take over. We have a much better chance at regulating our cortisol, leptin, and dopamine releases. Removing the provision for our flesh gives us a chance to formulate godly desires, just as Romans instructs us to do.

Instead of starving our bodies of nutrition and nourishing our sugar cravings, let's starve the cravings and nourish our bodies.

There is a lot of talk about discipline and motivation in the health world. It's great if you have discipline or feel motivated. That may begin your journey, but it won't sustain it. It's far better if you form a habit. Simple, easy habits, like keeping your home free of trigger foods and planning ahead for healthy snacks and meals, will ensure success when discipline ditches you and motivation melts. **Discipline eats motivation for breakfast. Habits eat discipline for lunch.**

Have you prayed for God to remove your sugar cravings, but they still keep controlling your choices? Do you feel like a spiritual failure? I've always craved Jesus. For most of my life, I craved sugar. Not anymore. I would never have thought it possible. But it's true. For so long I thought I was weak spiritually when the real culprit was my chemistry. That knowledge freed my soul from so many layers of guilt. I knew I needed to do the work to clean out the cupboards, but at least I could release the burden of blame

I placed on my spiritual life for so long. I wasn't a bad person; I simply had a bad cycle of addiction in my brain.

I never thought I would see the day that I did not wrestle with a desire for sugary foods, but I pray my experience offers you a glimmer of hope for your own journey. The day I decided to detox and eliminate refined sugars from my diet, the hold on me began to weaken. It took a solid week of headaches, jittery nerves, and feeling lethargic, but by day seven I had renewed energy and less desire for sweets. By the end of four weeks, my palate had cleansed and I started to crave healthier foods. I didn't know there were people who actually didn't care about baked goods and who didn't feel tempted by a dessert menu, but now I am one of them. I don't want to live like the average American, overdoing it on sugar. Nor do I want to live like a mouse in a test laboratory. I want to live supernaturally.

Your God-honoring habits are sugar-high downers. They will keep you grounded when you get the notion to go in search of strawberry shortcake or white chocolate mochas. Satan will try to deceive you into believing that you are weak spiritually, but your health journey is likely more about your brain than your soul. As you detox your body, let the Holy Spirit detox your guilty conscience.

I believe God when He says He works all things for good for those who love Him. My friend and coauthor of several books, Wendy Speake, leads a yearly sugar fast. In her book on the topic, she writes, "We suffer spiritually each time we reach for a sugar high rather than the Most High." I wasted a lot of precious effort on my sugar addiction. There really is no high like the Most High. Wendy goes on to say that "when God sets us free from the strongholds in our lives, we're free to experience His strong hold."[5] As you eliminate refined sugar from your everyday life, you will no doubt feel the need to have it, but the struggle won't last forever. When we leave Lollipop Lane behind, we walk down a path of victory. At the end are all the good things that God has prepared for you to enjoy, and they are far sweeter than sugar.

Let's Pray

Dear Father, I'm addicted to sugar. I feel it deep in my brain where my chemistry keeps me hooked. I understand how my body responses have worked against my heart's desires. I need a reset. Break the stronghold of sugar in my life. I want to experience You, the Most High, more than my sugar highs. Thank You for using everything—including this struggle—for good in my life. In Jesus' name, amen!

twenty-two

When One Mistake Makes You Want to Quit

Jonathan sat down on the edge of his bed and removed his shoes. Sighing heavily, he didn't dance around the subject. He made a decision. He wasn't going to try anymore. Cursing himself, he lay down, punched his pillow, and sank into the oblivion of sleep.

After all, he had spent four weeks perfectly on track, eating proper portions and staying hydrated with water. Twice a week he managed to get down to the office gym to work out during his lunch break. And then, that morning, he found himself driving by his favorite donut shop on the way to work. He had overslept, and instead of his usual breakfast of an omelet with spinach and avocado slices, he guzzled his coffee and headed out on an empty stomach. In his mind's eye, he would grab a hard-boiled egg from the office refrigerator, but he never got that far.

The car almost drove itself as it slid into the parking space in front of the bakery. Two jelly donuts later, Jonathan felt awful physically, but the real pain was in knowing he had made a big mistake. If he couldn't even make it past a month without giving in to temptation, then why bother heading into month two?

The feelings of defeat that Jonathan felt are common when we enter our health journeys. Many of us have an all-or-nothing mindset, and yet few circumstances in life lend themselves to perfection. Your personal health journey is one of them. Honestly, how often has an all-or-nothing mindset served you well? Journeys connote the idea that it's going to take a while, and it's going to have its fair share of bumps along the way. Miles will stretch before us with all their peaks and valleys, their miry bogs and scenic buttes. With this understanding, we are less triggered to veer off course when we stumble or struggle. If we expect to never stray from our eating plan or miss a day of exercise, we are tempted to throw in the towel when we do, and chalk up our desire to get healthy as unattainable.

Does this way of thinking even make sense? Is it logical?

What if Jonathan, sitting on the edge of his bed, gave himself grace? What if he acknowledged that he made a mistake, as humans often do, and then recommitted to his health plan? The Lord's mercies for us are new every morning and they never end (Lamentations 3:22–23). If He can show us mercy, surely we can offer it to ourselves.

Mistakes don't make us misfits—they make us human! **One meal, one choice to eat off plan does not erase a healthy lifestyle!** One poor choice doesn't negate the hundreds of good decisions Jonathan already made leading up to that moment in the donut shop. **The mistake is not the critical moment. The critical moment is *after the mistake*—the moment when you decide to either grow from your weakness or give in to it.** What if Jonathan took that mistake and turned it into a memory . . . and nothing more? Not a defeat. Not an ultimatum. A memory of a time he will be careful not to repeat. Suddenly, that mistake becomes an opportunity. Triggers are opportunities—if we choose to view them that way.

As a mom of four sons, I felt the delight of watching my kids take their first tentative steps as toddlers. They fell again and again.

They got up again and again. Such tiny people taking big strides toward growth. Never allowing the uneven ground or the hard knocks to keep them down. If we trip and stumble on the sidewalk, do we choose never to walk again for fear we may trip and fall again? Or do we become more aware of uneven ground? Do we give in to a life of stagnation, sitting in a chair for the rest of our lives, or do we see the value of walking and keep going? It's absurd to think we would give up a life of ever walking again simply because we don't always do it perfectly. And yet, we are willing to give up on our health, which has the potential for life or death, after one donut. Or one excessive meal. Or one week on vacation when we go off course. We decide to sabotage a potentially healthy future for the rest of our days because of a microscopic and momentary lapse. Perhaps it's time to renew our mindset.

> The critical moment is after the mistake—the moment when you decide to either grow from your weakness or give in to it

One of Jonathan's downfalls was driving past a donut shop without a new mindset and without a tool to help him replace his old pattern with a God-honoring habit. It's not his fault. Not really. He simply didn't know what to do when temptation beckoned. It felt like the car was driving itself, but really, Jonathan was simply not mindful of his actions. He allowed the moment of hunger—and the old feelings of desire—to overtake him. He began thinking about chocolate sprinkles on pink frosting and sugar-glazed donut holes. This habit of operating on autopilot must become who we once were, not who we now are.

Scripture is ripe with this concept:

> Therefore, if anyone is in Christ, the new creation has come: The old has gone, the new is here!
>
> 2 Corinthians 5:17

So how can we stay the course? Visualizing the new creation we are becoming is a great place to start. And I don't mean just physically. By now, we can see that our health journey is never just about food or dropping dress sizes. It's about becoming the best version of ourselves that we might become people who persevere, develop character, and abound in hope:

> Not only so, but we also glory in our sufferings, because we know that suffering produces perseverance; perseverance, character; and character, hope. And hope does not put us to shame, because God's love has been poured out into our hearts through the Holy Spirit, who has been given to us.
>
> Romans 5:3–5

In the aftermath of making an unhealthy food choice, we often feel ashamed. Hopeless. This is the very opposite feeling of what God longs for us to experience! After an unhealthy binge on garlic bread or chocolate fudge cake, I felt crestfallen. Instead of conviction, I felt self-condemnation. Condemnation is not from God. In my parenting book *Triggers*, my coauthor, Wendy Speake, and I longed to help parents ditch the voices in their heads that told them they were failures, ruining their children's lives when they yielded to frustrations. Satan is relentless in this messaging. Whether it's in parenting, our marriages, or our food journeys, his tactics rarely take new shape. In that first book, I wrote,

> Guilt defeats. Conviction catapults—towards spiritual growth and freedom! God always convicts us with a loving reproach that causes us to want to keep going in His strength and not in our flesh. It moves us forward toward growth in our spiritual lives, instead of backwards or inwards toward discouragement.[1]

If we are feeling guilt and discouragement, you can bet that is not of God. Let's not listen to that nonsense any longer. Instead, let us accept loving godly conviction and allow that to catapult us toward life to the full! That is what God longs for us to experience.

Jonathan forgot that he did not have to give in to the force of the temptation. As soon as he felt himself thinking about driving toward the donut shop parking lot, he had the option to replace that thought with a new one. You see, we are not victims of our circumstances, nor our temptations. God is the director of our steps, so let's not allow our emotions—or our hunger pangs—to have so much power! We have the privilege and honor of becoming a force for good in our own lives as we take full stewardship over our bodies.

Another tendency that often derails our good intentions is when an obstacle comes and we think that because things are hard, we made a mistake. And then worse, we allow that obstacle to stop us in our tracks toward progress.

Recently, I spoke with a client, Opal, who was about to begin her health journey with me. We had an excellent conversation about all the wonderful things she was going to gain by eating healthy and changing her mindset. I thought the call went great. And then she messaged me a few hours later. "I'm starting to panic!" she said. "My body is used to Chinese food! I eat a lot of rice and fried meats and vegetables. I'm used to making these things for dinner every night." Opal was a pillar in her large Asian-American family, where food was an important focus. Family meals were often full of carbs—and a lot of love! She wasn't sure she could go a day without wontons or chow mein noodles.

Now, I knew that once she got healthy and into a suitable BMI range, she could introduce healthy grains and enjoy leaner versions of her favorite foods again. And she knew that too. This wasn't really about chow mein. It was the fear that she had to be all or nothing in order to lose weight. It was either orange chicken and family and comfort and bonding, or lettuce and rejection and loneliness and isolation.

And that might be a possibility. Her family may turn their nose up at chicken salads instead of fried rice. So what? Do we really think that our families will not be happy for us as we try to better ourselves? Possibly. Will dinners become battlefields? They may. The question to ask is, *Is it worth it?*

Opal was stewing in the fear that she couldn't please her family and support her health at the same time.

One of her *whys* was being a good influence on her family. She expressed concern about their struggles with obesity and disease. Stretching before her was the opportunity to do all the things she longed for: creating longevity in her own life and helping those she loved to do the same. But when the rubber met the road, she wasn't truly ready to be the dominant force in her life. She gave that power to the wontons and her family members. She allowed the thought of being all or nothing to grip her with fear, resulting in panic.

We talked through the plan once more, and I reassured her that her family recipes would be there waiting for her in a few months. We talked through healthy alternatives to her favorites—things like cauliflower rice with shrimp, steamed dumplings, baked salmon with minimal soy sauce, and Chinese chicken salads. But more than anything, I longed for Opal to see that making choices to get healthy does not mean we live a life of all or nothing. Unfortunately, after only two days into her health journey, she quit. The process of detoxing was just challenging enough that she didn't want to continue.

Detoxing and getting healthy is hard. Living with obesity and disease is hard. We all must choose our hard. Going through a challenge does not mean we are making a mistake. It may very well be the best thing that could happen to us, if we are willing to see it through to the other side. If we are going to be a force for good in our own lives, we must be willing to consider that when the hard moments come, it does not mean we made a mistake and we should quit. It means we are transforming, allowing ourselves to put on a growth mindset that does not give in—we persevere, just as God would have us do!

Maybe you made a mistake today—a choice you regret. Perhaps you have set yourself up for failure with an all or nothing mindset, or perceived challenges as a signal to stop trying to reach your health goals. Blunders are not blockades to a better you. The better you lives on the other side of that obstacle. Get up and over it, leaping forward as you soldier on toward victory. The Bible assures us that nothing is impossible with God. The only "all in" mentality we need to have is not expecting a seamless transformation, but being committed to persevering toward our goal.

Let's Pray

Lord, I don't want to view my mistakes as reasons to quit on my health journey. I know You are long-suffering and want what is best for me. You never view me as a failure, so help me not to see myself that way. Thank You for giving me new mercies every morning. In Jesus' name, amen!

twenty-three

When You Are Downright Hungry, and Hangry Too

When mealtimes approach and my kids whine, "I'm hungry, Mom!" I'm quick to remind them that hunger is not always a bad thing. *Hunger* is not a dirty word. It's a sign—a signal that you are a human with needs. Hunger is a good thing because it alerts us that our bodies are doing their jobs, burning energy, and giving us life.

Hunger triggers can lead to bigger issues, however. When we are hungry, we can get into the habit of getting angry. Hunger plus anger leads to being "hangry." Testy. Moody. Less reasonable. We feel hunger, and we take it out on whoever is nearby. Viewing hunger as a positive feeling rather than a trigger that makes us hangry is a life-giving mindset switch. As Christ-followers, we can even allow the physical hunger pangs to turn us toward spiritual satisfaction.

Macki, a reader turned friend, messaged me. "I need help," she said. We first connected in a group for budding authors where I was giving a training on writing nonfiction books. Macki had read *Triggers* and was part of my launch team for *Marriage Triggers*, but now she was interested in the health plan I was using to keep healthy. We had spent time together face-to-face over the last year, so I knew she was in pretty good shape physically, but I could hear the desperation in her voice. She and her husband own and operate an impressive veterinary practice with dozens of employees, manage a small farm in Mississippi, and have three beautiful daughters who Macki homeschools full time. "I don't have time to eat, and my mood swings are not healthy for any of us," she shared. Macki admitted that she wasn't just hungry, she was hangry.

In Macki's case, she didn't need to lose weight, but her metabolism and blood sugar levels were making her feel exhausted, grumpy, and depressed. She didn't feel healthy because her body was releasing hormones that hindered her from feeling like herself. She loved her family and she loved Jesus, but she felt overcome by her reactions to triggers throughout the day.

It's not just Macki. Many of us experience the same thing when we are not keeping our blood sugar regulated by eating often enough. Once again, this food trigger can be partially explained with biology. When you haven't eaten in a while, your glucose levels drop and cortisol rises. The release of cortisol has been found to increase aggression in some people. One researcher notes that "low blood sugar may interfere with higher brain functions, such as those that help us control impulses and regulate our primitive drives and behavior."[1] When we are finished with a meal, our digestive system moves into action.

Specialized contractions called the migrating motor complex (MMC) sweep up undigested food, which is a process that takes around 130 minutes. The final phase of the MMC is regulated by a hormone called motilin. Motilin-controlled contractions cause the rumbling in our stomachs and coincide with hunger pangs in humans. Another hormone implicated in hunger control is ghrelin. In mice, ghrelin activates neurons called agouti-related peptide (AgRP)-expression neurons in the hypothalamus region of the brain, which tell us that we are hungry. These neurons are the control center for hunger.[2]

This cycle works in our favor if we eat something every two to three hours and keep our blood sugar stable. But like Macki, most of us are erratic in our eating habits. Macki joined me and a small group of moms to work on her health, increasing her hydration, eating smaller healthy meals or snacks every two to three hours, and getting more rest at night. The change was dramatic and swift. Her energy levels soared, and she finally felt like she had a handle on her emotions. Fueling her body regularly allowed her to have the energy she needed to do all the good work God has entrusted her to do. But she needed to put structure in place by engaging with me as her health coach, and planning ahead by preparing healthy snacks and meals to ensure healthy habit formation.

If you, like me, get hangry when you are hungry, there are practical things like the aforementioned we can do to help ourselves, but not all "hanger" relates to blood sugar. It's helpful to know what's going on inside our bodies so we can combat some of our weaknesses, but so much of this journey away from unhealthy patterns is about holiness. **Understanding the science behind our triggers doesn't eliminate the spiritual forces at work within us.** It's also not a free pass or excuse for ugly behavior.

If it's true that Jesus satisfies all our longings, and the fruit of the Spirit—like patience and kindness—is part of our soul's makeup, then it's also true that we are not at the mercy of cortisol or any other hormone. He who created cortisol is not subject to it, and having been made in God's image, neither are we. We can feel cranky and still be kind! The difference will be in breaking the pattern of impulsivity and moodiness by mindfully nurturing self-control.

How hungry are you to break the pattern of anger and frustration in your life? Do you yield to weakness instead of allowing the strength of the Almighty to rule your heart and tame your triggers? Psalm 84:2 says, "My soul yearns, even faints, for the courts of the

LORD; my heart and my flesh cry out for the living God." I want to hunger and thirst for righteousness more than ravioli or rum punch. I want my desire to respond in a God-honoring way to overpower my body's tendency to react in hanger. When I make a bad choice, I don't want to bring others down with me by being easily angered.

When I wrestled for self-control in my own health journey, I reached a point where my cries for holiness drowned out my yearnings for hamburgers. Only then did I have the power through the Holy Spirit's help to think before I spoke and pause before I plunged into angry reactions I would regret.

I believe that many of us reading this book want to make that shift, but we are overwhelmed. We aren't taking care of our bodies externally, so we have less emotional stability to respond gently and biblically when we are interrupted by our kids or cut off by a large truck on the highway. In my early years of parenting, when I struggled the most with anger, it's no coincidence that I also struggled with my weight. I allowed the demands of parenting three young children to crowd out my time with the Lord, and it showed.

Luke 6:45 says, "A good man brings good things out of the good stored up in his heart, and an evil man brings evil things out of the evil stored up in his heart. For the mouth speaks what the heart is full of." We can put all the right things into our body, but if we are not filling our hearts with truth and love, our mouths will reveal what we are really made of. There are many thin, healthy people whose hearts are obese with evil. As much as I meditate on my body and believe in self-care, that is no substitute for soul-care. **Embarking on our health journey is the perfect time to make provisions for the purification of our hearts and minds as well as our bodies.**

Ephesians 4:26 says, "Be angry and do not sin . . ." (ESV). **Even when your emotions run high, you don't need to stoop low or give in to temptation.** Proverbs 19:11 reminds us that "good sense makes one slow to anger . . ." (ESV). Once again, taking a moment for a "holy pause" before we open our mouths allows us time to cool down and exercise self-control. Good sense has a chance to swallow our hanger whole.

Sadly, some of my hanger came from my own guilty conscience. I was mad at myself for eating junk, and then I let junk flow from my mouth. Innocent bystanders got my mouthful. **When my mood swings got the best of me, I missed out on God's best *for* me.** Instead of being a blessing to my family, I was a bear to live with.

In those moments, a God-honoring habit is to ask yourself, "What is the root of my irritability, right now?" or "Will what I'm about to do or say help the situation or hurt it?" If we recognize we are simply mad at ourselves—not at our kids—that is the moment to pray and ask God for His grace. That is the moment to remember that we are not condemned when we yield to one more handful of popcorn. We confess our sin and receive a cleansed heart, free from guilt and shame.

Part of healing my body required healing relationships. I had to apologize to my family for letting my anger and insecurities color my vision. I needed to acknowledge the sin of both my gluttony and my rude spirit. It's not a coincidence that when I started to cleanse my body of fake food while simultaneously asking God to cleanse my heart of false beliefs, the journey became a joy instead of a juggernaut in my life.

Matthew 5:6 offers us this promise: "Blessed are those who hunger and thirst for righteousness, for they shall be satisfied" (ESV). Feast on *God's Word* and your hanger won't have the *last word.*

Let's Pray

Lord, I feel angry a lot. My mood swings are getting the best of me. I want Your Word to control my emotions, not food. Help me to eat healthy meals that regulate cortisol and give my body and mind a chance to stabilize. Thank You, Lord, for forgiving me and cleansing me from all unrighteousness. In Jesus' name, amen!

twenty-four

When You Feel Ashamed

They tried to shame her, all right. She was caught in adultery, and they were ready to stone her. The crowd of religious leaders, feeding on the drama of the moment, dragged her to Jesus. The intensity of the life-or-death moment does not rattle Him. They question Jesus, asking Him what they should do with the woman, no doubt trembling and clothed in nothing much more than her shame, at His feet. On one side, justice clamors for her death. On the other, compassion says, "Let any one of you who is without sin be the first to throw a stone at her" (John 8:7). You can almost hear the stones slip from their fingers and thud to the ground as they silently acknowledge that they too are guilty of sin. One by one they trickle away until only Jesus is left:

> "Woman, where are they? Has no one condemned you?"
> "No one, sir," she said.
> "Then neither do I condemn you," Jesus declared. "Go now and leave your life of sin."
>
> John 8:10–11

Perhaps you are familiar with this evocative story from the Bible, and you find Jesus' compassion beautiful. You may even feel confident that the woman did just what Jesus said. She gathered her skirts, dusted off the dirt on her hands, and turned over a new leaf, ready to take Jesus up on her second chance. But then you picture yourself, and by the time you finish this paragraph, you are ready to put a cloak of shame around your shoulders to hide your muffin top and head back to the cookie jar for one more Girl Scout cookie. Maybe we can even accept that Jesus forgives us, but we can't forgive ourselves.

Shame is defined as "the painful feeling arising from the consciousness of something dishonorable, improper, ridiculous, etc., done by oneself or another."[1]

That's exactly how I felt after finishing a third bowl of Lucky Charms. There is a difference between being bad and doing bad things. When shame floods our minds, we can't differentiate between the two very well. There wasn't much that felt "lucky" about my behavior, and I definitely did not feel "charmed." Three bowls of anything always felt "dishonorable," "improper," and "ridiculous." For me that translated to "I am dishonorable." And "I am improper." And "I am ridiculous."

What we often miss is that shame makes us self-centered. *I. I. I.* Our thoughts turn inward on ourselves, but the self-conscious life is not the selfless life that God wants us to live. **Pride doesn't care if we think too highly of ourselves or too lowly of ourselves; as long as we focus on "me," it's done its job.** All that emphasis on self was making me miserable.

> Pride doesn't care if we think too highly of ourselves or too lowly of ourselves; as long as we focus on "me," it's done its job.

The shame we feel about our bodies and the behavior that leads to being overweight doesn't just crush us spiritually; it acts as a perpetrator to even more shame-induced exploits. There is a recording in our head that says, "I'm already a failure, so what does it matter if I have another slice of pizza?" **Shame whispers defeat to our hearts, and the stench of it is tinted with the sulfur of Satan's breath.** Our food triggers are missiles launched from our enemy to weaken and defeat us. Satan does not want strong bodies or strong souls fighting the good fight—and shame is one of his favorite tactics for achieving his mission.

Compare that to what we know from Scripture. Satan will point his finger at you, but God's loving hand will embrace you and point you toward hope. God tells us that in the future, we will stand before Him to answer for our earthly lives. He says, "On that day you will feel no shame because of all your deeds by which you have rebelled against Me" (Zephaniah 3:11 NASB). Did you hear that, dear one? I have said before that there is a difference between conviction and condemnation. Satan will condemn you. He will gloat over your feelings of guilt, hoping you will wallow in the crevices of the land mines he has set for you. But God will lovingly convict you. He will remind you that He created you for good works and that He has chosen you because you are precious to Him, just as you are—there on the ground in the shadow of your accusers or standing at the kitchen sink with a rainbow-colored milk mustache.

He will lift you up and point you toward the heights of hope. Allow that conviction to catapult you toward a life where you "go and sin no more."

The night before I began my health journey several years ago now, I told my husband that I was looking forward to a healthier and happier reflection in the mirror, but more than anything, I was praying that the shackles of shame I felt around my ankles would break once and for all. It was my shame and sin that motivated me the most. I was tired of feeling bad about myself. Every time I opened the closet, I felt like a modern-day Eve, trying to hide behind clothes that didn't truly fit. As a Christ-follower, that attitude didn't fit either. Shame and embarrassment are two of the hindrances Paul urges us to throw off so we can run the race and win the prize! In order to "go and sin no more" (John 8:11 NLT), one of the first steps for many of us will be to cleanse our hearts before we clean out the wine cellar. I began with this prayer:

> *Lord, I confess that I have been an overeater and that I have not had self-control. I'm sorry. I know You love me, just as I am, and that You forgive me. I feel ashamed of myself and I don't want to feel that way anymore. I need Your help, Lord. Thank You for cleansing me from all sin. Help me to overcome my food triggers, one at a time, and grant me victory. In Jesus' name, amen!*

Shame shrinks with every word of confession and confidence in Christ. You are not a failure or a terrible person. God gave His Son for you because you are valuable to Him! God doesn't base His love for you on how you look or what you can or cannot do. His love is pure. Unconditional. Available! Jesus would leave the ninety-nine to find the one lost sheep. Your life matters. You matter. Your health journey matters. Along the way, you will not journey alone.

> What man of you, having a hundred sheep, if he has lost one of them, does not leave the ninety-nine in the open country, and go after the one that is lost, until he finds it? And when he has found it, he lays it on his shoulders, rejoicing. And when he comes home, he calls together his friends and his neighbors, saying to them, "Rejoice with me, for I have found my sheep that was lost." Just so, I tell you, there will be more joy in heaven over one sinner who repents than over ninety-nine righteous persons who need no repentance.
>
> Luke 15:4–7 ESV

As you choose a healthy eating plan, ban refined sugars from your kitchen, and dust off your jogging shorts, you may very well see the wolf in sheep's clothing darting past your kitchen window on occasion. He will lurk about from time to time in the form of food triggers, tempting you off track. His aim will be to lure you into believing that a bad choice makes you a bad person. He will attempt to slip the shackles of shame around your shrinking ankles. When those times come, and they will, look to your Shepherd. He stands beside you all the while, leading you, one victory over temptation at a time, toward the safety of His embrace. He does not condemn you. He rejoices over you! The path He guides you on is one littered with the shackles of others who have gone before you, each one a reminder that there is hope for you too.

Let's Pray

Lord, I confess that I have been an overeater and that I have not had self-control. I'm sorry. I know You love me just as I am and that You forgive me. I feel ashamed of myself and don't want to feel that way anymore. I need Your help, Lord. Thank You for cleansing me from all sin. Help me to overcome my food triggers, one at a time, and grant me victory. In Jesus' name, amen!

twenty-five

When You Are Addicted to Food

'll admit that food consumed me for many years. Thinking about
food, shopping for food, creating events so I could eat food were
big parts of my life. In my ancestry, addiction is part of our lineage. Alcohol, drugs, shopping—the hints of unhealthy patterns
and, in some extreme cases, the lives cut short as a result—are all
part of my unfortunate family legacy.

Growing up, I thanked God that I had not run the gauntlet of
this generational stronghold, but I was ignorant. My addiction to
food was simply more acceptable in our culture. The impact of it
was less obvious to those around me until the mirror forced me
to see what others already could. Eighty excess pounds packed on
slowly, but by the time I owned my reality, I was dangerously close
to becoming another broken branch in my family tree.

As a health coach, I have heard similar stories over and over
again. Ariel made two drive-through runs every day. Nathan
couldn't go to sleep without first enjoying his evening wine
and cheese. Brenda's morning didn't really begin until she had

completed her morning bagel run. Jacob rewarded his long days with midnight chip binges. Some of us know we are addicted to sugar, alcohol, or even just the comforting routine of eating and drinking our favorite beverage, but some of us haven't truly acknowledged the food habits that are harming our health.

I'm not sure what it was about the day I reached out to my friend for help, but I came to the point where I knew I couldn't change on my own. The Holy Spirit had convicted me for many months about my unhealthy patterns, but I had to come to a point where I stopped ignoring those whispers to my heart. Perhaps you are at that point right now. You are tired of the excuses you have been making. Weary from feeling discouraged and afraid that you will never change. Your addiction to food has a chokehold around your neck and you are ready to pry off its pudgy fingers, one at a time, and once and for all.

You have seen the impact of sugar addiction in chapter 21, and the accompanying chemical response of dopamine, but even salt and carbohydrates can trigger the pleasure centers of our brains. One doctor explains the behavior angle of food addiction:

> Compulsive overeating is a type of behavioral addiction meaning that someone can become preoccupied with a behavior (such as eating, or gambling, or shopping) that triggers intense pleasure. People with food addictions lose control over their eating behavior and find themselves spending excessive amounts of time involved with food and overeating or anticipating the emotional effects of compulsive overeating.[1]

For a long time, I prayed about my addictive food triggers. I wondered, *When will I be released from this struggle? Does God see me in this mess, and will He help me?* As I read through the Bible, over and over again I see impossible situations where God is faithful to deliver His people. More than that, God is not immune to how we feel in the midst of struggling with our food addictions and temptations:

For we do not have a high priest who is unable to empathize with our weaknesses, but we have one who has been tempted in every way, just as we are—yet he did not sin. Let us then approach God's throne of grace with confidence, so that we may receive mercy and find grace to help us in our time of need.

Hebrews 4:15–16

Is it possible to live without being a victim of our cravings? Does God understand our weakness? Will He help us overcome it, finally? Yes. Hebrews assures us that we can approach God with confidence, and that He will give us mercy and grace to help us in our time of need. On that day when I decided to make lifestyle changes, I came to a point where I recognized that God would do His part. I had to do mine.

What does your part look like today? This next hour? Picture yourself for a moment as you approach your next meal. What is on your plate? Who prepared it? Who went to the store and bought the ingredients? Was it you? If not, who gave the person serving you permission to plate your food? Was that you? Whose hands are lifting the fork? What is your part in what goes into your body and your mind? Until we see the reality of our eating patterns and fully acknowledge them, we cannot own our lives or master our addictions.

Yale University's Rudd Center for Food Science and Policy offers these questions to help us unveil whether we may be addicted to food or display unhealthy patterns. Do you

End up eating more than planned when you start eating certain foods?

Keep eating certain foods even if you're no longer hungry?

Eat to the point of feeling ill?

Focus on not eating certain types of foods?

When certain foods aren't available, do you go out of your way to obtain them?

The researchers also suggest we examine the personal impact on our relationships. Do you

Eat certain foods so often or in such large amounts that you eat instead of work, spend time with the family, or enjoy recreational activities?

Avoid professional or social situations where certain foods are available because of fear of overeating?

Have problems functioning effectively at your job or school because of food and eating?[2]

My answer to each of those questions was *yes*. Yes, I often overate. I often felt sick after eating. I often felt shame and avoided relationships because of my obesity. I avoided gatherings, events, and activities because of my unhealthy patterns and body image. Yes. Yes. Yes!

The day I began my new health journey, I had to say yes to something new. If you struggle with food, you will need to do the same. Together, we can now say yes to God's mercy. Yes to God's grace. Yes to His help. You and I get to answer the question of whether or not we believe we can change. We get to answer the question of whether or not our future will be one of victimization or vanquishment. I pray your answer, too, is yes.

Yes to being in control of who plates your food.

Yes to eating fruit, vegetables, lean protein, healthy fats.

Yes to making a grocery list and sticking to it.

Yes to your health.

Yes to your why.

Yes to your future.

While alcoholics can live without alcohol and abstain from drinking, food addiction requires us to learn to manage how to eat to live instead of eating to die. Food is necessary for survival. The accessibility of our drug of choice means that exchanging unhealthy patterns for God-honoring habits will make all the difference. Just because we must still eat doesn't mean we can't abstain from trigger foods—and trigger restaurants! There is no reason to make things harder on ourselves. Some of my trigger foods I committed to eliminating entirely from my diet were soda, chocolate, French fries, bread that was not whole grain, cow's milk, and artificial sweeteners. I also decided not to go to drive-throughs until I had a handle on my unhealthy patterns.

This journey away from addiction is not all about what we can't have. Focusing on what we think we are missing instead of what we are gaining won't help us. Making a list of what we get to have instead is a healthy mindset habit. Here's mine:

I get to eat delicious fruits and vegetables.

I get to learn new healthy recipes.

I get to have better skin and organ function by drinking sixty-four ounces of liquid every day.

I get to have an increased quality of sleep at night.

I get to avoid diabetes.

I get to avoid high blood pressure.

I get to avoid high cholesterol.

I get to have more energy.

I get to increase my longevity.

I get to have a better quality of life as I age.

I get to wear clothes I have always wanted to wear.

I get to feel more confident that I am in control of my choices.

I get to be an example to my kids.

I get to be in photographs again.

The spiritual battle over our food triggers is real. We may be overweight, but we are malnourished. **The only thing worse than a malnourished body is a malnourished soul.** None of our addictions are life sentences. I pray that my own life will serve to give you hope that if I can do it, so can you. Romans 15:13 says, "May the God of hope fill you with all joy and peace as you trust in him, so that you may overflow with hope by the power of the Holy Spirit." You don't have to wait to be hopeful. Yes, when the scale moves and your doctor tells you that you can stop taking blood pressure medicine, hope will rise. But hope and peace are available to you right now. God is the source of hope and peace as we trust in Him, and that is my prayer for you.

Some of us may need to receive counseling and extra support to overcome our food addictions. Like me, some of us will find a healthy plan to follow with the support of a coach and like-minded community. All of us have the opportunity to say yes to a life without food addiction. Know that God sympathizes with your struggles. I do too. Hebrews 4 reminds us to turn to God with confidence, that He will give us what we need when we need it. It may be that this book in your hands is part of His answer to your prayers for help. He will always do His part. Today you can do yours.

Let's Pray

Dear God, I'm ready to do my part. I'm ready to own my life and my choices. Father, I trust You to be my strength when I feel weak. This has been an unhealthy pattern for a long time, so now it's time to leave it behind. Thank You for giving me another chance to be an overcomer. This addictive behavior is in my past, but I now look forward to a healthy future. In Jesus' name, amen!

twenty-six

When You Feed Your Emotions

Jillian, a mom running a business from home, was eighteen pounds closer to her weight-loss goals when her septic tank backed up into their family camper while they were on a much-needed vacation. "My first thought, when the black sewage water began to rise, was *I want a cupcake*!" We were on a video chat talking about her recent month on the plan, and I could tell this was a critical moment for her. "But then I asked myself *why?*" She said, "No! Don't eat a cupcake, that's stupid! I don't even like the way they taste anymore!" In that moment, she could easily have given in to her emotions, but instead she made a thoughtful choice. Jillian had an opportunity to revert to her unhealthy pattern of feeding her emotions, but when the flood of sewage brought the flood of emotions, she made a better choice, and we can too.

Emotional eating is one of the most common reasons we overeat. To this day, it's still my biggest food trigger. Yes, I've learned to stop, challenge, and choose. I've practiced the habit of thinking

185

before eating over and over again. But even now, I don't always win. Life can be so very difficult, can't it? Pain overwhelms, and we need just a moment, just a touch, of immediate relief. Allowing the flood of feelings is too big a burden to bear. Loaded baked potatoes, chocolate chip pancakes, and five-layer lasagna take the edge off when we feel like we are about to go over the cliff.

The Institute for the Psychology of Eating says, "When people self-diagnose and say, 'I'm an emotional eater,' what they're saying is, 'I am doing this unwanted eating behavior that's driven by these unwanted feelings that I don't like.'"[1]

I'm certain that every emotional eater knows that the food is not going to fix the fear, the sadness, or the loneliness. But in the moment, its lure hooks us in. We are susceptible and vulnerable, and if we have not begun to practice healthier responses to food triggers, we are ill-equipped to resist. C.S. Lewis writes, "Without the aid of trained emotions the intellect is powerless against the animal organism."[2] Animals, by nature, rely on their instincts for survival. They operate in a reactionary way.

My son Quade loves to use a little red laser beam to play with our new kitten. All around the floor the light dances, and Miss Matilda is quick to pounce every time. She does not engage her thinking brain because as adorable as she is, she's not all that smart. She doesn't have the capacity of a human brain to observe, access, process, and make an intelligent decision about the temptation in front of her. As soon as she takes the leap, she comes up empty. But we are not kittens, are we? We have the ability to operate from a place of strength and mindfulness.

The automatic pattern of self-soothing with food has been a long-standing one for many of us. It's been an automatic reactionary behavior that relies on instant gratification but ultimately gives way to long-term guilt. This unhealthy pattern steals both our emotional health and our physical health. The emotions come, the trigger food is accessible, and we are sitting ducks, channeling our inner Miss Matilda.

It won't always be easy to replace emotional eating with a God-honoring habit. I want to acknowledge the emotions you feel and perhaps the ones you don't even realize are there, guiding you toward an insatiable solution. If, like me, you have been in the habit of yielding to your emotions, this is the day we begin to test them:

> Test everything; hold fast what is good.
>
> 1 Thessalonians 5:21 ESV

God's Word is useful for every aspect of our lives. If we got into the habit of practicing this one verse from 1 Thessalonians on our health journey, our lives would change dramatically. The moment of sadness is the moment when we get to demonstrate whether we believe God has given us the fruit of self-control.

That's the moment of truth. Triggered moments are testing moments.

In the center of the emotional storm, we will either spin out of control or self-regulate. **Emotions are not gateways to gluttony. They are portals for progress.** By questioning them, just as Jillian did when her house went from a place of refuge to a place filled with refuse, we become our own advocates on our health journey. She didn't peel a wrapper when the frustration hit her. She tested her impulse by asking herself why she wanted a cupcake. Instead of plunging into the temptation, she reasoned with herself that eating her emotions was not a smart move—nor would it satisfy her.

God tells us to "hold fast to what is good." Have you made progress on your health journey? That's good! Hold fast to it! Are you beginning to focus on your *why* when difficult days come in waves? That's good! Hold fast to it! Have you started drinking more water or sticking to the items on your grocery list? That's good! Hold fast to it!

Our emotions are designed to serve us, not enslave us. Everywhere we look, we see people being led by their emotions. Think back to one of your biggest regrets. Were emotions involved? Have you made some choices in life where you followed your emotions straight into a pit or a problem? I sure have! That's because our emotions are volatile. They don't always offer us a picture of reality. They talk to us very loudly when what we really need is calm and quiet to sort things out.

Emotions want us to act in the now when God encourages us to consider our ways before moving to action. They tell us that the guy in the car in front of us is a total jerk and we should blare our horn at him to teach him a lesson, when maybe he simply made a small mistake because of a tweaked rearview mirror. Our thoughts and emotions are the overflow of the condition of our hearts. They will either steer us in a good and godly direction, or they will become a roadmap to a dead end.

Let's imagine for a moment that we are settled around a cozy fire in the great outdoors. The music of the night is punctuated with the call of frogs and the buzz of fireflies. We sit in a circle with red-and-green plaid blankets tucked around our legs and steaming cups of coffee in our hands. The smell of pine trees is pungent and nostalgic. You are safe. Secure. Nowhere to go. Nothing to do. Just be.

What do you feel right now? What emotions have been lying under the surface? Which feeling has been too painful to acknowledge? How long have you tried to subjugate it?

There are many good ways to process our emotions. Eating to numb them is not one of them. **Feel what you feel, and don't numb it with a meal!** Let's decide to stop doing that, here by the fireside. Toss any emotion that is not serving you into the flames along with the unhealthy pattern of emotional eating. Your emotions are not more influential than your God. Don't be afraid of experiencing the force of your feelings. **Emotional hunger originates in our hearts, so feeding our stomachs will always leave us empty.**

There was never a day where I woke up and said, "Amber, when did you decide to be sixty pounds overweight?" The pounds packed on one at a time, one mismanaged emotion at a time. And they weren't all bad emotions; I ate when I was happy too! That's what

188

patterns do. They become so intrinsic to our lifestyle that we don't even realize the damage they are doing until we can't strap the airplane seat belt over our lap or fit into our favorite jeans.

My friend and mentor Nick LaValle remembers the shame and embarrassment he felt when he had to exit the roller coaster while his kids enjoyed the ride without him. After a failed attempt to sit in the seat, he was asked to meet the rest of his party at the exit. He will never forget the shame he felt as he walked away from the ride. That moment became the turning point for Nick. His troubled marriage and financial struggles were an emotional feeding ground. These new emotions forced him to accept his reality. Over the course of a year, he joined his wife, Kiersten, and learned to manage his emotional eating. A passionate Christ-follower, Nick committed to inviting Jesus into his journey. He lost one hundred pounds and now pays it forward as a world-changing leader on our coaching team. If it wasn't for Nick and Kiersten, I would not have begun my own health journey. Their willingness to manage their emotions with healthy habits has impacted thousands of others, including me. They are a perfect example of taking something good that God designed—our emotions—and using them to make a difference in the world.

> Emotional hunger originates in our hearts, so feeding our stomachs will always leave us empty.

Dealing with our primary emotions in a healthy way eliminates the need to deal with secondary emotions that come with emotional eating.

We are dejected over a broken relationship, so we eat.

We feel sad when our friend hurts our feelings, so we eat.

We rejoice over a huge breakthrough at work on a project, so we eat.

We are fearful about a diagnosis, so we eat.

The pressures of life press in, you got it—we are triggered to eat.

Our emotions have an important role in our lives. Food has an important role in our lives. Reframing our minds about the God-given gift of emotions helps us welcome feelings into our everyday experiences without using them as vehicles for harming ourselves by misusing food. **When the roles of emotions and food are placed in proper order, losing control of our eating becomes a habit of the past, not our future.**

Strong emotions bring up many fears within us. If we face the pain of our troubled marriage, we are sure our hearts will break into a thousand pieces. The feelings of betrayal from your best friend still bewilder you. The layers of protection around your heart have served to protect you from being betrayed again, but they have also formed a barrier from forming new authentic friendships. The many years of infertility have taken their toll and, even though you long to be content, comparison is stealing your joy. Your verbally abusive childhood has created such a strong need for justice in you that you never cut anybody any slack, and now your own adult children want nothing to do with you. Food has fettered your fears for a long time.

If we let them rise to the surface, what will happen to us?

First John 4:18 says, "There is no fear in love, but perfect love casts out fear" (ESV). Your emotions stem from imperfect experiences with imperfect people. That is the fallout of the fall. Trouble is Adam and Eve's legacy, but had we been in their animal-skin shoes, we would have done the same. Jesus reminds us that in this world, we will have trouble. He urges us to "be of good courage," for He has overcome the world (John 16:33 DARBY). Our earthly experience is not to avoid emotions; it's to view them in the light of heavenly promises. God is love and He loves you. Perfectly. Let that feeling be the one that reaches your heart and satisfies your deepest longings.

The day I woke up and had enough of my unhealthy lifestyle was the day I had to give my emotions to the Lord. It was the day I traded my fears for His love. It was the day I decided to believe that my emotions would not kill me, but my obesity would.

It turns out that experiencing my emotions—the good, the bad, and the ugly—has actually enriched my life and made me a better person. I know that Satan would love to use our emotions against us—against our own bodies to manipulate and destroy us. I grew tired of letting him use me against myself. When I made the choice to eat mindfully, not emotionally, I became more thoughtful, compassionate, and equipped to handle problems in a way that solves issues instead of exacerbates them.

My health journey has not just impacted my health. It has enriched my relationships and brought me closer to the Lord in ways I never knew were possible. That's what emotions do when we don't eat them. They serve us in the way God intended, so that even the ones that Satan may have intended to harm us are for our good.

Let's Pray

Dear God, Your love for me is perfect. I'm afraid that my emotions will be too painful to deal with, but I trust You to carry me through as I deal with them instead of bury them. I long to be free from the emotional drama I'm experiencing and the cycle of emotional eating. Thank You for being my Rock and my Redeemer. I put my faith in You to heal and restore me. In Jesus' name, amen!

twenty-seven

When You Are Fixated on the Scale

My son hid my scale from me," my client Brooke said with a laugh. She knew it was a good thing. Every day she was checking her weight, monitoring her progress. And every day her emotions bounced around with every bounce of the needle. She was just starting out on our health plan, but the struggle was real. Her fixation on the scale stemmed from an unhealthy pattern in her past that she wanted to overcome.

Is being at a healthy weight an indicator of overall health? Yes. Does the scale help us navigate our progress? Sure. But there are plenty of valuable non-scale indicators of healthy progress we may be missing out on.

One of the greatest joys of making progress on our health journeys is all the happy surprises we experience along the way. I remember the confusion I felt when my scalp began to heal just a few weeks into my own journey. I had been plagued with painful psoriasis for years, and all of a sudden, it was disappearing. I didn't put two and two together at first. It was a delight to realize that detoxing my body from sugar and processed foods wasn't just affecting the number on the scale, but also my overall health. My confusion led to celebration soon enough!

So how often should we be weighing ourselves? The importance of shifting our mindset away from the scale is foundational to our overall success long-term. Some studies show that weighing yourself daily is the best way to go, as those who do tend to catch themselves sooner if their healthy habits begin to slip. But for other people, the scale controls their emotional well-being. In those cases, it's better to weigh just once a week or even monthly.

One of my clients does not weigh herself at all. Her fixation with the scale was so strong that she simply ditched it and focused on how she felt and whether her clothing felt looser. Our needs for weighing ourselves will be as varied as we are. Each of us is on our own unique journey and should do what is best for whatever season we are in at the moment. Becoming a person who is disciplined to make those discerning choices is the process that allows us to honor God in this journey. If that means asking your spouse to hide the scale, then do it!

Non-scale victories (NSVs) are some of the most valuable areas to focus on when losing weight. They often catch us off guard. One of my clients told me that she was walking along, minding her own business, when her skirt fell down a little and she stepped on it. Thankfully, it didn't fall off!

Recently, my client Reese sent me a message. She was nine months into her health journey and only three pounds away from a hundred-pound weight loss. "We are headed out to Park City, Utah, for our family ski trip next week, and I just can't wait to see what skiing with 97 fewer pounds feels like! I think it has been about 20 years since I have been around this weight. I'll send pics from the mountain," she wrote. Skiing with 97 fewer pounds meant nearly four hundred pounds of pressure released from her joints. Can you imagine?

Another client, Callie, was only two weeks into her health journey when her son fell ill and she had to cancel her fortieth birthday
bash with friends and family that she had been looking forward to
for months. "Normally, things like this would have made me want
a glass of wine or to bake some chocolate chip cookies (and eat
like five of them). But I have been sticking to the plan. Not even
desiring a glass of wine! Woo-hoo!" she told me. Woo-hoo is right!

Yet another client told me she could see her stomach over her
chest when she is in the down-dog yoga pose, and another can
now paint her own toenails! One client noticed that a stubborn red
patch of skin on her ankle had vanished. Another said he couldn't
believe how much he enjoys discovering new wines and healthy
dishes that are on his plan when he goes out to eat with his wife.
Several clients recently shared how the inflammation in their bodies has disappeared, and another called me in tears because she
went from an A1C blood glucose level of 10 to 6.1 in a matter of
months. She was just shy of no longer being considered a diabetic!

Guy and I went shoe shopping after we reached our goals. Every
shoe I tried on felt floppy and way too big. I couldn't figure it out.
I grabbed the shoes and hurried over to the men's department.
Guy saw me coming and said, "Honey, I'm wearing a size smaller
shoe!" I stood there bewildered. "It's because we lost weight!" he
exclaimed. Finally, it dawned on me. I couldn't believe that my
weight loss actually changed my feet! Sure enough, I tried on a
size smaller, feeling a little bit like Cinderella, and it fit!

All the ways we experience the blessings and benefits of being
healthy are numerous. We rob ourselves of the gift of overall health
when we narrowly focus on a number. Each of these clients had
days when the scale went up or down, but by focusing on the NSVs,
they were able to stay on track.

I remember the days before I started my health journey. I had
allowed my weight and my body to take up a lot of my brain space,
and I was tired of it. Every time I put on a sweater, I spent time
fluffing it out to see if it would hide my rolls of fat. I searched for

the chair at the back of the room so the women at my Bible study class couldn't see my rolls spill over the waistband of my pants. I spent my mornings trying to contour my face with makeup in a useless effort to resurrect cheekbones and minimize my double chin. I spent hours with doctors trying to get to the bottom of how to heal my psoriasis, arthritis, and achy back. Once a month I landed in the emergency room for fluids and pain medication to get me through a migraine. Wasted time. Wasted money. Wasted energy. Wasted mindset.

Here I was, a Christ-follower, knowing my life was but a vapor and that I needed to make the most of it, but I was fixating on the scale and on all the secondary problems related to my weight. Romans 14:17–20 says,

> For the kingdom of God is not a matter of eating and drinking, but of righteousness, peace and joy in the Holy Spirit, because anyone who serves Christ in this way is pleasing to God and receives human approval. Let us therefore make every effort to do what leads to peace and to mutual edification. Do not destroy the work of God for the sake of food.

Paul is addressing the squabble among believers in the early church who were at odds with one another about whether they could still eat the foods they were accustomed to eating under their former religious practices. In essence, Paul informs them that they are missing the bigger picture. They were laser-focused on the rule and missing out on the relationships they were meant to nurture as a body of Christ. They were growing surly over food when they should have been growing in peace and joy, seeking to build one another up.

Though the circumstances are different, I felt a bit like those early believers when I considered what food was doing to my mindset. I was thinking way too much about things that didn't have any eternal value. I was wasting my time and efforts on superficial things and elevating food and its impact on my life over the good things God wanted me to experience. To sit in a Bible study and be thinking more about how uncomfortable I felt trying to cross my legs than how I might offer a word of encouragement to the women around me was a wake-up call.

If we are fixated on anything besides Jesus, we are fixing for disappointment. It's in Christ alone that we find security, value, purpose, and hope. In fact, when our eyes are on the scale in such a way that our entire mood and choices are dictated by it, we lose sight of what the future holds. The moment of truth at the scale clouds our vision for the better things God wants to reveal to us. First Corinthians 2:9 says, "'What no eye has seen, what no ear has heard, and what no human mind has conceived'—the things God has prepared for those who love him." There is so much good awaiting us! Let's not miss it!

> If we are fixated on anything besides Jesus, we are fixing for disappointment.

How do you feel after you weigh in on the scale? Disappointed? Delighted? Discouraged? Determined? Doubtful? Disgusted?

It's normal to feel something, of course. It's what we do with those feelings that makes the difference.

Is the pattern of allowing the scale to rule your heart hindering your ability to focus on things that truly matter? Do you spend a lot of time thinking about your weight? Remember my client Brooke? When the scale messes with your emotions, you may need to ditch the scale. **Don't give the scale too much power over your emotions. If it ruins your day, walk away!**

Commit to identifying more of your non-scale victories. Celebrate them! More than anything, remember that we were not created for our stomachs; our stomachs were created for us! We are the boss! We get to tell it what's what, not the other way around. The scale is one tool in your toolbox. Don't give it more influence over you than it deserves. Make the main thing the main thing—living a life that honors God, fixing our eyes on Him, who is far more worthy of our focus than the scale.

Let's Pray

Lord, thank You for revealing so many victories to me along my health journey. I don't want to be fixated on the scale, but on You. Help me to appreciate each new blessing of getting healthy. I want to be a person whose emotions are used for good, not to harm me. It feels good to make progress, and I praise You for it. In Jesus' name, amen!

twenty-eight

When People Compliment You but It's Hard to Accept

A ll she knew was that she wanted to lose weight and feel better. Sure, looking better would be nice, but Nora wasn't too concerned about her appearance at the start of her journey. She was thrilled to finally be losing the weight that was bogging her down both in mind and body. After a few months, people started to notice. A little on the shy side, Nora wasn't prepared for the reactions of others. In a way, the extra pounds had acted as a comfortable barrier between herself and others, but now the protection was being removed and she felt like a spotlight was focused on her success. Colleagues, friends, and family started to compliment her, making her feel even more exposed and vulnerable.

Tricia stumbled over her words every time someone told her she looked like she had lost weight. After just a few months into her health journey, she had lost thirty pounds—a dramatic and noticeable change. Her friends were happy for her, but every time she tried to accept the compliments, she felt a surge of guilt. "It makes me feel conceited," she said. My beautiful friend Christine told me that she has learned to say thank-you when someone compliments her, but it's still hard for her to accept. "My perception and beliefs about myself do not match the compliment. It feels incongruent, and as if it's not correct, not that I don't deserve it." Others shared with me that they automatically shoot down the compliment, qualify it, or dismiss it. Many readers have shared that they constantly feel unworthy of compliments and have even rebutted with sarcasm as a defense mechanism.

Exchanging unhealthy patterns for God-honoring habits isn't just something we do. It's something we believe. There is an epidemic of unworthiness that men and women are facing. Some of it is habitual and some of it is spiritual.

Tricia wasn't in the habit of receiving compliments, so when they came, she wasn't in the habit of accepting them either. As Christine shared, the praise and attention we may get from others doesn't always feel true of us.

I spent many years obese, so when I lost sixty pounds in just under six months, I hadn't fully accepted my new reality. When I looked in the mirror, I could see what others saw, but in my head, I was still that obese girl who felt extremely uncomfortable and unattractive. My mind had not caught up with reality! The compliments contradicted my own self views.

> Exchanging unhealthy patterns for God-honoring habits isn't just something we do. It's something we believe.

This trigger is more than superficial, however. Our inability to accept the affirmations of others lies deeper in our souls. I believe that the way we think of ourselves has been whispered to us by our enemy who wants to devour us and defeat us emotionally.

On one hand, we can graciously acknowledge that God did something good when He knit us together in our mothers' wombs.

We can also accept that beauty is in the eye of the beholder. God made us to be attracted to beauty and to appreciate it in all its varied forms. On the other hand, we can become prideful and self-centered. Full of ego and placing too much importance on appearances. They are two very different things.

Tricia, who told me she felt conceited by acknowledging the kind words about her from others, is one of the sweetest and least conceited people I know. I believe that many of our issues with valuing ourselves come from a good place. We want to be humble. We desire to be selfless. We want to bless others. Nobody wants to be seen as an egotistical monster, and yet those who are concerned about that are typically not the egotistical monsters!

The flip side of the coin is that when we compliment someone, our desire is to affirm and uplift them, and it's deflating when they reject what we say. I know I come away feeling a bit let down in my effort to be kind to them. Receiving the praise of others is a way for both of us to feel blessed!

Imagine if Rahab had not been bold enough to believe that she wasn't just a worthless, discardable prostitute. When Joshua's spies entered her house scouting the land that had been promised to the Israelites, she hid them and boldly asked for what she wanted:

> Now then, please swear to me by the LORD that you will show kindness to my family, because I have shown kindness to you. Give me a sure sign that you will spare the lives of my father and mother, my brothers and sisters, and all who belong to them—and that you will save us from death.
>
> Joshua 2:12–13

In her culture at the time, she could have been made to feel like a wallflower, hesitant and self-conscious, but instead, she boldly highlighted her own act of kindness and asked for what she wanted. She accepted that these men believed in her ability and trusted her. Singlehandedly, Rahab rescued the spies by lowering them down a wall via rope and, in the end, spared her entire family from certain destruction. Furthermore, she would be listed in Jesus' lineage! Rahab was no wallflower.

In the New Testament, an angel approaches Mary, a young teenager betrothed to Joseph, a humble carpenter. The angel tells her she is "favored by the Lord." Luke 1:29 says that Mary "was startled by what the angel said and tried to figure out what this greeting meant" (GWT). Surely the affirmation about her did not match up with the view of herself, a poor young girl with nothing special to single her out. Mary questions the angel's meaning, and after explaining to her that she was going to become pregnant and mother the Savior of the world, she does not shy away from the honor. Instead, Mary answers, "I am the Lord's servant. Let everything you've said happen to me."

In Psalm 139, the psalmist affirms the God-honoring habit of acknowledging good things about ourselves. He says, "I will give thanks to you because I have been so amazingly and miraculously made" (v. 14 GWT). In verses 17 and 18, we see how highly God thinks of us:

> How precious are your thoughts concerning me, O God! How vast in number they are! If I try to count them, there would be more of them than there are grains of sand.

If God has more precious thoughts about us than we could count, how could we not accept the affirmations and goodwill of others? Over and over again, God's value in His people is clear. Even when we were sinners, at our worst, Christ died for us. We are valuable beyond measure to Him. If we don't believe that about ourselves, we are calling God a liar. That's not territory I'd step into. Accepting the compliments of others is a good step in the right direction in affirming and honoring God for the good work He did in creating us and equipping us with various talents and abilities. Learning to accept our own bodies and graciously embrace the compliments of others is an important part of embracing our God-given value.

I know, for some of us it still feels conceited to embrace the compliments of others. The definition of *conceit* is "Excessively proud of oneself; vain."[1] So let's test it out. Does this definition really describe you? I'm betting it doesn't. So release the fear that others will think this of you. If you had such a big head, they probably wouldn't be complimenting you in the first place. They'd be avoiding you!

It's true that man tends to look at the outward appearance while God looks at the heart (1 Samuel 16:7). That doesn't equate to putting ourselves down or feeling like we have to be ugly or unattractive to others in order to be humble. Even Esther went through many months of beautification treatments in order to be selected as the future queen. She used her looks—and her position—to save a nation.

When someone compliments you, take it at face value and say thank you. Move on in gratitude. Be thankful that they see the evidence of a lot of heart work and hard work to reach this transformation.

Accepting compliments is another way that our health journey transforms us into stronger people. When we say thank you, we are practicing thankfulness. Take a moment to acknowledge that you reflect God's good work. A heart filled with gratitude has very little room for pride or conceit. It's a holy paradox. By embracing the goodwill of others, we don't set ourselves on a pedestal. It's just the opposite. We have the opportunity to grow in true humility. I can't think of a better way to live our lives than from the posture of gratitude. Take each kind word as an opportunity to reflect on all God has done to transform your body and your heart along this journey, and return to Him the praise.

Let's Pray

God, You did a good thing when You made me. Help me to believe that! Help me to value myself as You do. I want to be gracious and receive compliments from others. Help me to stay humble and kind and to enjoy the goodwill of friends and family who see a change in me. In Jesus' name, amen!

twenty-nine

When Self-Care Is Not a Priority

My dad woke up in the dark, put on his suit and tie and a dash of musky cologne, and left the house for work every morning. His hair was black, slicked back like Elvis Presley, whom he resembled. I'd watch his shiny-coated head dip into his yellow Dodge Colt as he left for work. It would be dinnertime before he returned. I looked forward to that front door opening every single evening. To this day, my father is one of my favorite people. He worked hard to provide for us, and he never complained about it. It was he who sat next to me at bedtime and read books, night after night, instilling in me a love for stories that shaped much of who I am. I can't ever remember a time when he asked for anything for himself. He was happiest when we were happy.

I learned a lot about contentment from my dad, but a piece of me always felt sad that he didn't do much for himself. I knew he had hobbies he enjoyed, and so often he sidelined them to participate in activities for us kids or serving others at church or working longer hours to please his boss. One thing that has always been true of my father, however, is that he made his health a priority. Even now, at seventy-five years old, he has a nightly strength-training exercise routine, and he eats right—and it shows.

He may have passed on a love for books, but I didn't pick up on his commitment to taking care of oneself. The demands of being a stay-at-home mom are hard to grasp until you have experienced it. That's when I began to gain weight, slowly but surely, over the years of having kids and raising them. It's natural to nurture and pour out our lives for our kids, but I came to a point when everything I had emotionally and physically was devoted to everything and everyone else but me.

And I was happy to do that. Until I wasn't. Then that day came when I felt spent. Weary. Exhausted. Depleted. I didn't even have the margin of time to acknowledge how drained I was until my health problems—and my mood swings—began to speak louder than my responsibilities.

Three years ago, I took a baby step toward a big-girl moment of advocating for myself. One of my favorite things to do is sit in a massage chair at a spa and get a manicure and pedicure. It had been ten years since I made that a priority for myself. Once a month, every month since then, you can find me with my eyes closed among the hum of a busy nail salon as I sit back and let my nail technician, Wanda, work her magic. As a mom of four sons, I choose as much pink bling to decorate my digits as possible and enjoy every minute of my two-hour escape.

Having that monthly ritual is just enough to remind me that I am not just an extension of my kids or my husband. I exist too. Eventually, I took the step of investing in healthier foods and prioritizing my time each week to work with my health coach. Because I had already taken a small step to protect a couple of hours once a month for a pedicure, it was that much easier to make my health journey a priority too!

The idea of self-care sounds abrasive to our ears. It's a little bit like fingernails on a chalkboard. We cringe when we hear that term. Conditioned to think of a life well lived as one of sacrifice and service to others, we have missed the truth that we can't do that well if we are not first taking care of ourselves.

The World Health Organization describes self-care as "what people do for themselves to establish and maintain health, and to prevent and deal with illness. It is a broad concept encompassing hygiene (general and personal), nutrition (type and quality of food eaten), lifestyle (sporting activities, leisure etc.), environmental factors (living conditions, social habits, etc.), socio-economic factors (income level, cultural beliefs, etc.) and self-medication."[1]

Do we honestly think that God would not want us to give attention to our health, prevent disease, have good hygiene, eat nutritious foods, develop an active lifestyle, and foster a healthy environment? Consider again 1 Corinthians 6:19–20:

> Do you not know that your bodies are temples of the Holy Spirit, who is in you, whom you have received from God? You are not your own; you were bought at a price. Therefore honor God with your bodies.

I understand that getting my nails done is not a necessity, but the mindset behind taking time to care for ourselves certainly is. You may not ever get in the habit of a weekly massage, but the minimum priority of self-care should be our overall health, striving for a healthy weight for your body frame, and supporting our cardiovascular system with exercise. Our bodies are "temples of the Holy Spirit," and every food trigger we overcome is our way of giving Him the honor and respect He is due.

One of my favorite stories in the Bible is about Elijah. On the run for his life after being used by God in miraculous ways, he was weary to the point of death. God, in His kindness, sends an angel to restore him:

All at once an angel touched him and said, "Get up and eat." He looked around, and there by his head was some bread baked over hot coals, and a jar of water. He ate and drank and then lay down again. The angel of the LORD came back a second time and touched him and said, "Get up and eat, for the journey is too much for you." So he got up and ate and drank.

1 Kings 19:5–8

God knows we are only human. In the same way that Elijah needed nourishment and rest for his body, so do we. It's especially tender to see how the angel of God acknowledged that the journey was "too much" for him. Perhaps that is how you feel today. You love God and you love others. But the foreseeable future feels like too much. You are depleted and now it's time to be refreshed and restored. Even Jesus left us this example as He often went away to a quiet place to pray and spend time with His heavenly Father.

For some of us reading this chapter, we are still squirming at the idea of prioritizing ourselves. **Being selfless is not the same as being self-punishing.** If I'm in the hospital recovering from a heart attack, I'm not going to be much good for anyone! If I'm driving all over town, taking kids to playdates because I want them to learn that relationships add value to their lives, but never make time for my own friends, then my messaging is hypocritical. Like my dad, I know men tend to sacrifice a lot for their families, but in my experience, it's mothers who especially struggle to do things for themselves. God did not design us to become absorbed in the lives of others. He created each of us with a specific purpose and with supernaturally designed talents and abilities. That's because we matter to God! **Your needs matter just as much as your child's do because you are a child of God!** If we say we can't get healthy because we are too busy with parenting, then we better be prepared

> Being selfless is not the same as being self-punishing.

to look them in the face and tell them that they are the reason we are obese. Can you imagine? It's a horrifying thought, and yet that is essentially what we are doing when we allow anything or anyone to become an excuse for our unhealthy patterns.

Over the years, I've seen firsthand how prevalent a lack of self-care is for most of us. There are 10,080 minutes in a week, and yet clients struggle to make time for a fifteen-minute call with their health coach to get critical support on their health journey. Just sixty minutes a week to get outside and enjoy a hike feels like a luxury. Parents will spend hundreds of dollars on sports equipment for their kids or even on a daily Starbucks run for their spouse on the way to work, but they won't spend a little extra on healthier grocery options. No wonder our nation is spending billions of dollars and is facing a crisis of preventable disease and mental health issues.

Mark 12:30 says, "Love the Lord your God with all your heart and with all your soul and with all your mind and with all your strength." We are not separate from our souls. Our bodies are made up of heart, soul, mind, and flesh. We are to love God with all our being, including our physical bodies. Paul, in Romans 12:1, exhorts us to present our bodies as "a living sacrifice" to God. That's one way we actually worship God! Sacrificing the pleasure-inducing patterns of eating things that do not support our health or longevity is one way we can actually honor God!

Take a bubble bath, call a friend, get good sleep, drink plenty of water, read your Bible, take the dog for a walk, buy lean protein and low-carbohydrate vegetables, book a massage, take regular showers, spend five minutes taking deep cleansing breaths, dust off the elliptical machine, or simply learn to sit down at the table to eat your meals. Colossians 3:12 instructs us to clothe ourselves with kindness. How can we be kind to others and be so unkind to ourselves? It's incongruent and not consistent with God's desire for our well-being. We don't have to be a statistic. Now is the time to exchange those unhealthy patterns for God-honoring habits. Do you need permission? I'm giving it to you. But more important, God has given it to you.

Let's Pray

Dear God, I have not been taking care of myself. I have allowed everyone and everything to have more importance in my life than my own health. I'm sorry. No more excuses. Today I commit to making room for self-care, knowing that You love me and want me to be my best. Thank You for placing great value on my life. In Jesus' name, amen!

The Journey Continues

Reaching your goal weight and getting healthy isn't the end of your health journey. It's the start to truly living! Read these last two chapters with confidence and joy as you reflect on your path to wellness and embrace the blessings of living life to the full.

thirty

When You've
Reached Your Goals

ongratulations! All that hard work on your health journey
has paid off! You are enjoying the euphoria of reaching
your goals and living a new life with the good habits you
have put into place. Take a moment and relish it!

But . . . now what?

Recently, someone asked me for statistics on how many people
maintain their weight loss after reaching their goals. While numbers abound, the bottom line is this: One hundred percent of those
who continue to eat healthily and follow the habits of health that
they have used to transform their bodies will continue to maintain
and be healthy. One hundred percent of those who neglect healthy
habits, binge on junk food, live a sedentary lifestyle, and abandon
self-control will not maintain their health. The choice is yours!
Still, transitioning to maintenance is a time to renew your sense
of purpose and accomplishment by reflecting on your successes
at overcoming your triggers and looking to the future.

In the weight loss stage, you were burning more calories than
you were consuming, so now is the time you may need to increase

your healthy calories to stabilize your weight. A good health coach or your doctor can advise you.

This stage can feel a little scary! You have enjoyed seeing the scale move lower and lower, and now it's going to stay where it is. This new healthy habit of weight loss must now shift to a healthy habit of maintenance. **Our goal has been to reach the parameters of health guidelines, and now our goal will be to stay there.**

There are lots of good things to look forward to once you have embraced a healthy lifestyle. One of my clients has recently taken up bike riding, and another brought home a trophy from a motocross competition thanks to his renewed energy and stamina. The greatest joy for me when I overcame many of my food triggers was knowing that I achieved something I doubted was possible. **God really did show up so I could shape up!** Maintaining this way of life is evidence that your faith has carried you through. That's an awesome spiritual confidence booster right there.

You and I have now awakened to possibility. We get to look for other areas of our lives where we can conquer stubborn fears or step out of our comfort zones. Some of my clients begin new hobbies, change careers, take the leap to stay home with their kids, or become health coaches themselves to pay it forward. When you realize that your unhealthy patterns no longer dictate your choices, your potential becomes limitless!

Think back to the person you were before you began your health journey. What were your biggest food triggers? Which of your old, unhealthy patterns were most grievous to you? Psalm 119:59 says, "I have considered my ways and have turned my steps to your statutes." You see, this journey away from food triggers' unhealthy patterns has not been about food alone. The journey has been spiritual. Each of us, as we enter a maintenance period, can say with the psalmist, "I have considered my ways." One by one, we have uncovered the roots of our food issues and have exposed them in order to overcome them. Again, like the psalmist, we can say we have "turned my steps to your statutes."

God-honoring habits are a reflection of your willingness to obey God by stewarding your body and allowing nothing to take root in your life except that which will refine you and allow you to bear the fruit of the Holy Spirit. Our aim is not perfection. It's a willingness to yield to the perfecting work of the Holy Spirit, which does not end when the scale hits a certain number. We all know that this journey will have its missteps. The difference now is that you have proven to yourself that you are, indeed, an overcomer. Your missteps did not end your journey. They were simply part of it.

The imagery of God our Father as a gardener in John 15:1–2 has always delighted me. He "cuts off every branch in me that bears no fruit, while every branch that does bear fruit he prunes so that it will be even more fruitful."

Your old patterns were like gnarled leaves deadened and lifeless. Each time you faced a food trigger and worked through it, God's hand has been there, removing the parts of your mindset and behavior that have not been serving you in your journey. You did not face your food triggers alone. God is not absent from your life. **You need not simply muscle through when God is there to carry you through!** Let that truth keep you immersed in your healthy lifestyle.

God says that when we remain in Him, He will remain in us. He describes himself as the vine and we are His branches, connected, alive, and nourished by Him (John 15). We are not able to bear fruit of any kind—including achieving optimal health through our new habits—unless we keep clinging to the vine.

> You need not simply muscle through when God is there to carry you through!

Can we lose weight? Sure. But bearing fruit and growing spiritually as a result are only possible when we do so from a place of obedience and worship. Continue on this garden path with God as your companion.

So how do we achieve lifelong health and wellness now that we have reached our goals? God says that "apart from me you can do nothing" (v. 5). God uses all things in our lives, our struggles, and our triumphs to further our relationship with Him. In His benevolence, He shows us His willingness to help us each day as we seek to honor Him with our bodies.

In the same passage from John, God lovingly says, "Whatever you ask in my name the Father will give you." I begin every day of my life by taking time to pray and acknowledge that I need God to help me. Proverbs 16:3 says, "Commit to the LORD whatever you do, and he will establish your plans." Do you want to experience the blessing of obedience? Do you want to remain successful in your health journey? Commit it to the Lord!

A lack of confidence was one of my unfortunate byproducts of being obese. Like me, you may not have become accustomed to this new you just yet. That's okay. Put your confidence in the Lord. He has already promised you success when you remain in Him and commit your way to Him.

As a healthy man or woman, you are not the norm in our society anymore. Statistically, we know that most people are overweight and obese. But not you. You have leaned in to the supernatural strength of God to help you, and it has made you into something new. That's what God is in the business of doing. Second Corinthians 5:17 says, "Therefore, if anyone is in Christ, the new creation has come: The old has gone, the new is here!" It's likely that you may even look like a new person. Let your reflection be a daily reminder that we are still being made new spiritually. **One way or another we will be in maintenance. We get to decide what we want to maintain.** Unhealthy patterns? God-honoring habits? Enter this transition with a renewed commitment to God and to yourself. Be intentional to thank God for the good work He has done in you, and maintain a commitment to bearing fruit in every new season.

Let's Pray

Dear Father God, thank You for this new time of transition in my health journey. You have made me into a new creation both physically and spiritually. I want to stay connected to You and bear fruit in my life that has eternal value. I don't want to be afraid of gaining weight back. Help me to lay that aside and keep making my healthy choices. Thank You for being my hope and my help. In Jesus' name, amen!

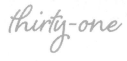

When You Need to Celebrate Your Victories

They took a mere six steps forward and stopped. After enemies had taken the ark of God captive, King David had a mind to bring it back to Jerusalem. During the initial attempt, the ark was placed on a cart for transport. In order to steady the ark, Uzzah, one of the men assisting the process, reached out and touched it—a fatal mistake.

The holiness and reverence for the ark had not been upheld. The mission was halted and for three months, the ark rested in the house of Obed-Edom. Eventually, David tried again. Hoisting the ark onto wooden slats to be carried this time, the men took a mere six steps, and with thousands to go, they stopped to sacrifice a bull and fattened calf. Early on in their journey of obedience, they paused to acknowledge how far they had come and their need for God's favor for the remainder of their journey.

As the ark of God made its way into the city of Jerusalem, "David was dancing before the LORD with all his might, while he and all Israel were bringing up the ark of the LORD with shouts and the sound of trumpets" (2 Samuel 6:14–15). There is no inhibition as David and his people celebrated this incredible victory and achievement. Their response was to delight in it and worship God through dancing and music.

At the end of my clients' first week on their health plan, I schedule a Zoom meeting to celebrate them. We call it a celebration call for a reason—there is usually a lot to celebrate! By eating clean and regulating their blood sugar, even in such a short window of time, most clients have experienced detox and are finally feeling an energy spike, sleeping better, and have become more mentally cognizant. Time and time again they describe a lift from their mental fog. They have also experienced a significant weight loss in that first week and, for many who have felt stuck for so long, it's a euphoric moment. We clap and beam with pride over their accomplishments and spend time talking about all the amazing healthy changes they have made over the last six days. Like King David, we take the time to pause, early in the journey, to thank God and rejoice over their victories.

If we don't come alongside our clients and celebrate them, they will go uncelebrated. They won't do it for themselves. We are not in the habit of celebrating our own successes, but this is an important part of our health journey. **When we acknowledge that we have made changes and overcome some of our most challenging unhealthy habits, we also have an opportunity to thank God for His help along the way.**

Celebrating even small victories affirms that God is helping us to leave the old self behind in exchange for the new creation He is making in us. Have you stopped mindlessly grazing on your kids' plates? Celebrate it! Did you finally drink sixty-four ounces of water today? Celebrate it! Take the stairs instead of the escalator? Celebrate it! Did you stop and think about the healthy options available before choosing a restaurant for your anniversary? Celebrate your marriage, indeed, but don't forget to celebrate your healthy habits! Did you stay on plan for a whole week? Celebrate it!

Experts say, "These moments of celebration make us pause and be mindful, and that boosts our well-being. According to social psychology researcher Fred Bryant, when we stop to savor the good stuff, we buffer ourselves against the bad and build resilience—and even mini-celebrations can plump up the positive emotions which make it easier to manage the daily challenges that cause major stress."[1] We already know that this journey has its high points and low points. Each time we celebrate a success, it strengthens our resolve for the next challenge. Every time we celebrate turning a corner, we gain momentum for the twists and turns along the remainder of the journey.

Celebrating is a healthy and godly habit, but the way we celebrate matters too. You don't have to throw a huge party for every victory in your life, but there are healthy ways to mark milestones in your habits and weight loss. Indulging in a high-calorie meal or polishing off a bowl of ice cream is not the healthy way to go. Celebrate by telling a friend of your accomplishment and enjoy their praise and affirmation. Take a break for five minutes to visualize the person you were before and who you are now, offering a prayer of thanksgiving to God for the transformation. Rewarding yourself with a day of golf or a spa day to rest and recharge after reaching a major goal is a healthy way to celebrate that also complements your healthy lifestyle. Buy yourself some new clothes or take a friend out for coffee. Celebrating in healthy ways supports your commitment to overcoming unhealthy patterns.

> Celebrating is a healthy and godly habit, but the way we celebrate matters too.

Most people in our lives will be eager to celebrate along with us, but not always. When King David entered the city, dancing before the Lord with wild abandon, some observed him with disdain:

> As the ark of the LORD was entering the City of David, Michal daughter of Saul watched from a window. And when she saw

King David leaping and dancing before the LORD, she despised him in her heart.

2 Samuel 6:16

David's own wife was repulsed by his display. She went on to tell him so to his face when he returned home from the festivities. Her words dripped with criticism, insinuating that even the slave girls would be influenced by his vulgar display, but David did not fall into the trap: "David said to Michal, 'It was before the LORD, who chose me rather than your father or anyone from his house when he appointed me ruler over the LORD's people Israel—I will celebrate before the LORD. I will become even more undignified than this, and I will be humiliated in my own eyes. But by these slave girls you spoke of, I will be held in honor'" (2 Samuel 6:21–22).

Even though his own wife did not understand his joy and accomplishment and what God had done for him and the people of Jerusalem, he was undeterred from her jealousy and unkindness. Michal could not rain on David's parade because he did not allow her to. Sometimes our journey will feel lonely, or we may be misunderstood by those observing from the outside, but let's be as stalwart as King David, ready and willing to celebrate the good work God has done in us and for us. Breaking free from the bondage of food and unhealthy thinking is a big deal, so it is okay to make a big deal about it! If others have been a part of your journey, celebrate them and their contribution as well. Most of us have had support from friends, family, and health coaches. If they have been there for the struggle, let's include them in the celebrations too.

One key element of celebrating is that it fills our hearts with the godly trait of gratitude:

Give thanks in all circumstances; for this is the will of God in Christ Jesus for you.

1 Thessalonians 5:18 ESV

And let the peace of Christ rule in your hearts, to which indeed you were called in one body. And be thankful. Let the word of Christ dwell in you richly, teaching and admonishing one another in all wisdom, singing psalms and hymns and spiritual songs, with thankfulness in your hearts to God. And whatever you do, in word or deed, do everything in the name of the Lord Jesus, giving thanks to God the Father through him.

Colossians 3:15–17 ESV

Every good gift and every perfect gift is from above, coming down from the Father of lights, with whom there is no variation or shadow due to change.

James 1:17 ESV

My own transformation process was lifesaving for me. When I was eighty pounds overweight, my spirits were low. Every day I felt like my obstacles got the better of me. I was thankful for the good things God had done in my life, but my health issues often overshadowed my feelings of gratitude. By eating healthily and becoming fitter, I experienced one success after another, day by day. **My perpetual series of victories left me in a state of perpetual gratitude.** Do you know what it's like to be around someone who feels stuck versus somebody who is filled with gratitude, hope, and joy? I said it before, but it was lifesaving for me—physically and spiritually! My confidence in the ability of the Holy Spirit to help me be victorious in other areas of my spiritual life began to flourish too. My health journey became the answer to my prayers for spiritual refinement and growth. Gratitude was the wind beneath my wings to help me soar.

The God-honoring habit of celebration is one most of us don't consider at first, but my prayer is that you will begin to relish life and every good work God does in you on this journey. You are an overcomer, my friend. In everything, we are called to be thankful. When our pants finally button, and our inflammation heals, and we pass right by the donut shop without a backward glance, we make every moment of our day one of praise and victory. You have exchanged your unhealthy patterns for God-honoring habits. There is no doubt in my mind that God is celebrating over you today. Remember that. Now go out and do likewise.

Let's Pray

Dear God, You are worthy of my praise! I am filled with grati-tude for every victory I am making in my health journey. Thank You, Lord, for showing me that nothing is impossible with You. I celebrate today's victories and I commit to exchanging my unhealthy patterns for habits that honor You. My heart over-flows with joy for each victory, big or small, and I offer You my thankful heart as an act of worship. In Jesus' name, amen!

Appendix

When You Have an Eating Disorder

While most of us deal with a number of issues on our health journey, those who struggle with eating disorders have a unique level of pain that is hard to bear and often requires professional help. These disorders are a deep-rooted struggle in the lives of countless men, women, and young people around the world. The secretive nature of these disorders makes it hard to find help. I'm convinced that every health journey will have its ups and downs, but for those of you who may have an eating disorder, I pray that this story from my dear friend Macki Smith, in her own words, will infuse your heart with hope.

The Lord is my strength and my song; he has given me victory.

Exodus 15:2 NLT

O ne of my favorite jobs in high school was working as a clerk for our local drugstore. I started out as a young preteen wrapping Christmas gifts during busy holiday seasons, and advanced my way up to running the front cash register. For a teenage girl, it was a dream job. And life working behind the local drugstore counter was always exciting.

Since I lived in the same small town for all of my childhood and saw the same people pick up their medications month after month, it was easy to grow friendships with our clients (since I knew most of them anyway). I would chat with them while ringing up their multivitamins or while showing them where to find the bottle of Extra-Strength Tylenol. We'd talk about the local football game last Friday night or where their kids were going for the summer. They'd tell me about their terrible migraine that kept them in bed for two days, how their two-year-old fell off the swing set and bruised his head, and how they lost all their baby weight by taking the diet pills we sold.

Through one of these simple conversations, I decided to try diet pills for myself to drop a few pounds. To me, they seemed to be just a "simple" appetite suppressant. And for an insecure, self-conscious girl who wanted to lose a mere ten to twelve pounds, diet pills seemed like the quick lose-weight-fast fix I needed.

The weight came off slowly at first, but after a few months, I was down to a coveted size 2. Finally, I could wear those jeans that snugged my hips in all the right places. And when other people started complimenting my weight loss, I was determined never to regain those extra twelve pounds again.

Although on the outside I appeared skinny, on the inside, I felt lousy because I was afraid to eat. The diet pills suppressed my appetite so much that I wasn't hungry anymore. And when I did eat, I saw food as an enemy that made me fat. Because I feared gaining the weight back, I would only eat a little bit each day. Eating too little made my energy levels bottom out and weakened my immune system. That year I stayed sick most of the time. I even had the flue and relapsed from it three times.

And yet, despite being the unhealthiest I'd ever been, the compliments about how great I looked kept rolling in. For months I stayed in the vicious cycle of taking diet pills, not eating enough, and staying sick.

Thankfully, God had a plan to wake me up and broke me of those chains of bondage. That summer I worked away from home as a camp counselor. There, God convicted me about what I had done to my body, and I realized that instead of harmlessly dieting, I had unintentionally developed a full-blown eating disorder. After God's intervention, I never felt the internal pull to take diet pills and deny myself food again.

Unfortunately, my bad relationship with food wasn't over. As a young mom in my midtwenties, I developed food sensitivities that made me severely sick. Instead of looking at food as something to make me fat as I did as a teenager, I began to see food as something that would make me sick. I longed to eat and even gain a little extra weight, but everything I ate hurt my stomach. I also lost three pregnancies during this season, which I fully believe was because my body was not healthy enough to sustain them. Again, I lost a ton of weight, but this time unintentionally. And again, like before, the compliments came rolling in about how great I looked and how wonderful it must be to be so skinny.

On the inside I wanted to scream because I knew skinny doesn't equal healthy. Through a lot of nutritional research, changing how I ate, and listening to my body, I eventually fixed my gut, increased my strength, and got healthy again. And in the end, God blessed me with more babies.

Ironically, the times in my life when I received the most compliments about my body were also the times I was physically the unhealthiest. It's sad how our culture feeds us the lie that skinny must equal beauty and health.

These days, I'm a busy mom who needs superhuman energy to run a household, a business, and a farm, and now I simply view food as fuel for my life. What I put into my body directly affects how I feel. If I put junk in my body, don't exercise, miss my daily vitamins, and don't drink enough water, I feel awful. When I don't take care of myself and eat well, I also lack the energy it takes to sustain myself and take care of the ones I love most.

Although it's been a bumpy ride, food and I finally have a healthy relationship. Thankfully, I now embrace food and nutrition as avenues to health and healing. Also, daily I pray God continues to give me the strength and energy I need so that I can fulfill all of His purposes in store for my life.

Acknowledgments

For my world changers and hope dealers . . .

Tammie, if you had not shared, I would not have changed my lifestyle. Thank you.

Kiersten and Nick, I'm a better person, spiritually, physically, and professionally, because of you. You are leaders and you are friends, but most of all, you are family. Thank you for changing my life.

Jamil, it started with you. Thanks for the mind shift. I will be among your twelve, always.

Dr. Andersen, besides Jesus and my family, nobody has had more impact on my life than you. You gave me hope, and without that, not much else matters. I'm honored to be a part of your grander mission to help transform the world, one healthy habit at a time.

To my sweet Guy, Oliver, Quinn, Oakley, and Quade: The transformation I experienced was for me, but everything I do, I also do for you. I want my example to be a strong legacy for our family. It thrills me that you want to be healthy too! Thank you for embracing this lifestyle with me! Together, we will keep paying it forward. I love you!

To Sarah Pollie, Laura Kreitler, and Alle McCloskey: You beautiful friends have been pivotal in supporting my ministry of writing. My life would have had a void without you in it. I thank the Lord for you!

To my agent, Janet Grant: You are simply the best. Your example of professionalism and your ability to both calm me and propel me toward solutions is a gift. Thank you!

To my editor, Jeff Braun: It was a long time coming but worth the wait to work with you. You have championed me from the beginning of my writing career, and I will never forget it. Thank you for making me a better writer!

To my publisher, Bethany House: Thank you for this opportunity to share my gut-honest message with readers. I'm honored to be a Bethany House author, and I will treasure the experience, always.

Notes

Chapter 1 When Your *Why* Is Front and Center

1. Craig Hales et al., "Prevalence of Obesity and Severe Obesity Among Adults: United States, 2017–2018," National Center for Health Statistics Data Brief, no. 360, February 2020, https://www.cdc.gov/nchs/products/databriefs/db360.htm.
2. Amber Lia and Wendy Speake, Triggers: Exchanging Parents' Angry Reactions for Gentle Biblical Responses (USA: Same Page Press, 2015), 212.

Chapter 2 When You Feel Defeated Before You Start

1. Juliette Tocino-Smith, "What is Locke's Goal Setting Theory of Motivation?" Positive Psychology, October 23, 2021, https://positivepsychology.com/goal-setting-theory/.
2. "Losing Weight," Centers for Disease Control and Prevention, August 17, 2020, https://www.cdc.gov/healthyweight/losing_weight/index.html.
3. F. Scott Fitzgerald, *Tender is the Night* (New York: Scribner, 1995 edition), 239.
4. Marianne Schnall, "An Interview With Maya Angelou," Psychology Today, February 17, 2009, https://www.psychologytoday.com/us/blog/the-guest-room/200902/interview-maya-angelou.

Chapter 3 When You Are Bored

1. Rick Warren, *The Purpose Driven Life: What on Earth Am I Here For?* (Grand Rapids: Zondervan, 2002), 21.
2. John Steinbeck, *East of Eden* (New York: Penguin, 2003 edition), 46–47.

Chapter 4 When Your Clothes Don't Fit and You Can't Hide It

1. Anne Chisholm, "The Tale of an Ugly Duckling," The Daily Telegraph, June 5, 2006.
2. Riley, "What Do Swans Eat? (7 Foods to Feed These Beautiful Birds)," October 6, 2018, https://www.natureinflight.com/what-do-swans-eat/.

3. Luke Ward, "15 Fun Swan Facts," The Fact Site, accessed April 2, 2021, https://www.thefactsite.com/15-fun-swan-facts/.

Chapter 5 When You Lack Portion Control

1. Recommended calorie requirements depend on several factors, including age and activity level. See "Estimated Calorie Requirements," reviewed by Kathleen Zelman, MPH, RD, LD on August 18, 2008, WebMD, https://www.webmd.com /diet/features/estimated-calorie-requirement.

2. Alan Mozes, "Most Restaurant Meals Exceed Recommended Calories," Web MD, January 20, 2016, https://www.webmd.com/diet/news/20160120/most -us-restaurant-meals-exceed-recommended-calories-study#1.

3. U.S. Department of Agriculture and U.S. Department of Health and Human Services, *Dietary Guidelines for Americans, 2020–2025*, 9th edition, December 2020, page 4; available at www.dietaryguidelines.gov.

Chapter 6 When Your Doctor Tells You to Lose Weight Before It's Too Late

1. Northwestern University, "U.S. population on track to getting even fatter," ScienceDaily, www.sciencedaily.com/releases/2011/11/111116132920.htm, accessed April 3, 2021.

2. Mark É. Czeisler, Rashon I. Lane, Emiko Petrosky, et al, "Mental Health, Substance Use, and Suicidal Ideation During the COVID-19 Pandemic—United States June 24–30, 2020," Centers for Disease Control and Prevention, August 14, 2020, https://www.cdc.gov/mmwr/volumes/69/wr/mm6932a1.htm.

3. National Diabetes Statistics Report, 2020, Centers for Disease Control and Prevention, https://www. cdc.gov/diabetes/library/features/diabetes-stat-report.html.

4. "The Health Effects of Overweight and Obesity," Centers for Disease Control and Prevention, September 17, 2020, https://www.cdc.gov/healthyweight/effects/index.html.

5. "Weight Loss Benefits for Arthritis," Arthritis Foundation, accessed April 2, 2021, https://www.arthritis.org/health-wellness/healthy-living/nutrition/weight -loss/weight-loss-benefits-for-arthritis.

Chapter 7 When Others Sabotage You or You Sabotage Yourself

1. Jamil Frazier, *The Twelve Shifts: Your Superpowers for Creating an Invincible Life* (Story Chorus, 2020), 178.

Chapter 8 When Community Means Food

1. Czeisler, et al, "Mental Health, Substance Use."

2. Mayo Clinic Staff, "Friendships: Enrich Your Life and Improve Your Health," Mayo Clinic, August 24, 2019, https://www.mayoclinic.org/healthy-lifestyle/adult -health/in-depth/friendships/art-20044860.

3. "Osteoarthritis Can Increase Your Risk for Social Isolation: Research Summary from the Journal of the American Geriatrics Society," Science Daily, October 15, 2019, https://www.sciencedaily.com/releases/2019/10/191015171548.htm.

4. "Osteoarthritis Can Increase Your Risk for Social Isolation."

5. C. P. Herman, "The Social Facilitation of Eating or the Facilitation of Social Eating?" *Journal of Eating Disorders*, April 27, 2017, https://jeatdisord .biomedcentral.com/articles/10.1186/s40337-017-0146-2.

Chapter 9 When Losing Weight Is Harder Than It Used to Be

1. Amber Lia and Wendy Speake, *Parenting Scripts: When What You're Saying Isn't Working, Say Something New* (USA: Same Page Press, 2017), 81.

2. Moira Lawler, "5 Reasons It's Harder to Lose Weight With Age," Everyday Health, June 27, 2019, https://www.everydayhealth.com/weight/weight-gain-and -aging.aspx.

3. Lawler, "5 Reasons It's Harder to Lose Weight With Age."

Chapter 10 When You Want to Be a Couch Potato

1. Dr. Wayne Scott Andersen, *LifeBook Journal* (USA: Dr. A's Habits of Health Press, 2019), 332.

2. Alessia Santoro, "In an Emotional Holiday Ad, a Grandfather Lifts Weights Ahead of Christmas for the Sweetest Reason," POPSUGAR, December 14, 2020, https://www.popsugar.com/family/emotional-holiday-ad-with-grandpa-lifting -weights-video-48056723.

Chapter 11 When You Travel

1. "U.S. Travel Answer Sheet," U.S. Travel Association, accessed April 2, 2021, https://www.ustravel.org/answersheet.

2. Chef Chang, "Eating Out vs Cooking at Home—The 12 Statistics You Must See," Slice of Kitchen, May 17, 2019, https://sliceofkitchen.com/eating-out -vs-cooking-at-home-statistics/.

3. Andersen, *LifeBook Journal*, 114.

Chapter 12 When Losing Weight Is Easy for Everyone but You

1. Jonny James, "9 Short Stories About the Journeys of People You Admire," Better Marketing, September 16, 2019, https://bettermarketing.pub/9-short-stories -about-the-journeys-of-people-you-admire-6bbc1852a409.

2. James, "9 Short Stories."

3. Olivier Poirier-Leroy, "The Problem with Comparing Yourself to Other Swimmers," Your Swim Book, accessed April 2, 2021, https://www.yourswimlog .com/the-problem-with-comparing-yourself-to-other-swimmers/.

Chapter 13 When You Need Support from Someone Else

1. "How Social Support Can Help You Lose Weight," American Psychological Association, accessed April 4, 2021, https://www.apa.org/topics/obesity/support.

2. Tricia Leahey and Rena Wing, "A Randomized Controlled Pilot Study Testing Three Types of Health Coaches for Obesity Treatment: Professional, Peer, and Mentor," *Obesity*, vol. 21, 5 (2013): 928-934, https://www.ncbi.nlm.nih.gov /pmc/articles/PMC3484232/.

3. "Study Shows Health Coaches Effective in Helping People Lose Weight, Live Healthier Lives," American Council on Exercise, October 2012, https://www .acefitness.org/certifiednewsarticle/2892/study-shows-health-coaches-effective-in -helping-people-lose-weight-live-healthier-lives/.

4. Best Life Editors, "20 Science-Backed Ways to Motivate Yourself to Lose Weight," Best Life, December 28, 2017, https://bestlifeonline.com/science-backed -weight-loss-motivation/.

5. Frazier, *The Twelve Shifts*, 192.

Chapter 14 When It's the Holidays

Mark McIntyre, "C.S. Lewis on Christian Morality," Attempts at Honesty, May 7, 2016, https://www.mhmcintyre.us/c-s-lewis-christian-morality/.

Chapter 15 When You Hit a Plateau

1. Mayo Clinic Staff, "Getting Past a Weight-Loss Plateau," Mayo Clinic, February 25, 2020, https://www.mayoclinic.org/healthy-lifestyle/weight-loss/in -depth/weight-loss-plateau/art-20044615.

2. Often misattributed to Aristotle, but is in fact Will Durant, *The Story of Philosophy* (New York: Simon and Schuster, 2006 edition), 98.

Chapter 16 When You Eat Mindlessly

1. Alyssa Pike, "Snacking on the Rise: 2019 Food and Health Survey Results," Food Insight, May 31, 2019, https://foodinsight.org/snacking-on-the-rise-2019 -food-health-survey-results/.

2. WeTheTrillions team, "America's Snacking Habits Are a Burden on Public Health. Here's What We Are Doing About It," WeTheTrillions, February 9, 2020, https://www.wethetrillions.com/learn/blog/american-snacking-habits-are -a-burden-on-public-health-heres-what-we-are.

3. WeTheTrillions team, "America's Snacking Habits Are a Burden on Public Health."

4. Statista Research Department, "U.S. Eating Behavior—Statistics and Facts," Statista, December 1, 2020, https://www.statista.com/topics/1558/eating-behavior/.

Chapter 17 When Your Favorite Beverage Keeps Calling Your Name

1. James McIntosh, "Fifteen Benefits of Drinking Water," Medical News Today, July 16, 2018, https://www.medicalnewstoday.com/articles/290814.

2. "Sugary Drinks," The Nutrition Source, Harvard T. H. Chan School of Public Health, accessed April 2, 2021, https://www.hsph.harvard.edu/nutrition-source/healthy-drinks/sugary-drinks/.

Chapter 18 When You Are Stressed

1. Valerie Bolden-Barrett, "Study: 94% of US and UK Workers Report High Work-Related Stress," HR Dive, September 11, 2018, https://www.hrdive.com /news/study-94-of-us-and-uk-workers-report-high-work-related-stress/531905/.

2. Valerie Bolden-Barrett, "Workers With Overstuffed To-Do Lists Feel Overwhelmed, Not Organized, Study Shows," HR Dive, January 24, 2019, https://www.hrdive.com/news/workers-with-overstuffed-to-do-lists-feel-overwhelmed-not-organized-study/546622/.

3. Nicole Galan, "How Do I Stop Stress Eating?" Medical News Today, February 15, 2018, https://www.medicalnewstoday.com/articles/320935.

4. Katie Hurley, "Stress vs Anxiety: How to Tell the Difference," Psycom, September 7, 2020, https://www.psycom.net/stress-vs-anxiety-difference.

5. Joyce Meyer, Instagram post, August 6, 2020.

Chapter 19 When Negative Self-Talk Overwhelms You

1. Sarah Zielinski, "Secrets of a Lion's Roar," *Smithsonian Magazine*, November 3, 2011, https://www.smithsonianmag.com/science-nature/secrets-of-a-lions-roar-126395997/.

Chapter 20 When You Are Lonely

1. "What Happens in Your Body When You're Lonely," Cleveland Clinic, February 23, 2018, https://health.clevelandclinic.org/what-happens-in-your-body-when-youre-lonely/.

2. Jamil Frazier, Instagram post, November 24, 2020.

Chapter 21 When You Are Addicted to Sugar

1. Yuval Noah Harari, *Homo Deus: A Brief History of Tomorrow* (New York: Harper Perennial, 2017), 14.

2. Wayne Scott Andersen, *LifeBook Journal* (USA: Dr. A's Habits of Health Press, 2019), 320.

3. Anna Schaefer and Kareem Yasin, "Experts Agree: Sugar Might Be as Addictive as Cocaine," Healthline, April 29, 2020, https://www.healthline.com/health/food-nutrition/experts-is-sugar-addictive-drug.

4. Andersen, *Lifebook Journal*, 321.

5. Wendy Speake, *The 40-Day Sugar Fast: Where Physical Detox Meets Spiritual Transformation* (Grand Rapids, MI: Baker Books, 2019), 17.

Chapter 22 When One Mistake Makes You Want to Quit

1. Amber Lia and Wendy Speake, *Triggers: Exchanging Parents' Angry Reactions for Gentle Biblical Responses* (USA: Same Page Press, 2015), 212.

Chapter 23 When You Are Downright Hungry, and Hangry Too

1. "Is Being 'Hangry' Really a Thing—or Just an Excuse?" Cleveland Clinic, December 24, 2018, https://health.clevelandclinic.org/is-being-hangry-really-a-thing-or-just-an-excuse/.

2. "Is Being 'Hangry' Really a Thing," Cleveland Clinic.

Chapter 24 When You Feel Ashamed

1. Dictionary.com, https://www.dictionary.com/browse/shame.

Chapter 25 When You Are Addicted to Food

1. Jennifer Casarella, "Food Addiction," Web MD, July 17, 2020, https://www.webmd.com/mental-health/eating-disorders/binge-eating-disorder/mental-health-food-addiction#1.

2. Casarella, "Food Addiction."

Chapter 26 When You Feed Your Emotions

1. Marc David, "Emotional Eating: Here's What You Need to Know," Institute for the Psychology of Eating, accessed April 2, 2021, https://psychologyofeating.com/emotional-eating-heres-what-you-need-to-know-video-marc-david/.

2. C.S. Lewis, The Abolition of Man (New York: Touchstone, 1996), 35; quoted at https://www.cslewisinstitute.org/Men_without_Chests.

Chapter 28 When People Compliment You but It's Hard to Accept

1. "Conceited," Lexico, accessed April 4, 2021, https://www.lexico.com/en/definition/conceited.

Chapter 29 When Self-Care Is Not a Priority

1. "What is Self-Care?" International Self-Care Foundation, accessed April 2, 2021, https://isfglobal.org/what-is-self-care/.

Chapter 31 When You Need to Celebrate Your Victories

1. Polly Campbell, "Why You Should Celebrate Everything," Psychology Today, December 2, 2015, https://www.psychologytoday.com/us/blog/imperfect-spirituality/201512/why-you-should-celebrate-everything.

Amber Lia is an independent certified health coach who has been on her own transformative health journey. She has written several books, including *Marriage Triggers*, and coauthored the bestselling parenting book *Triggers*. A former high-school English teacher, Amber is a sought-after mentor for women and a regular contributing writer for The Better Mom. Amber and her husband co-run the faith-friendly production company Storehouse Media Group, and they live in Southern California with their four boys. For contact information and to learn more, head over to AmberLia.com.